101

ESSENTIAL TIPS

Yoga

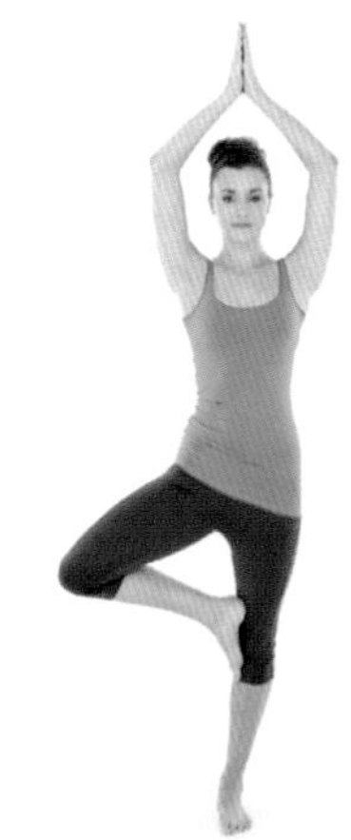

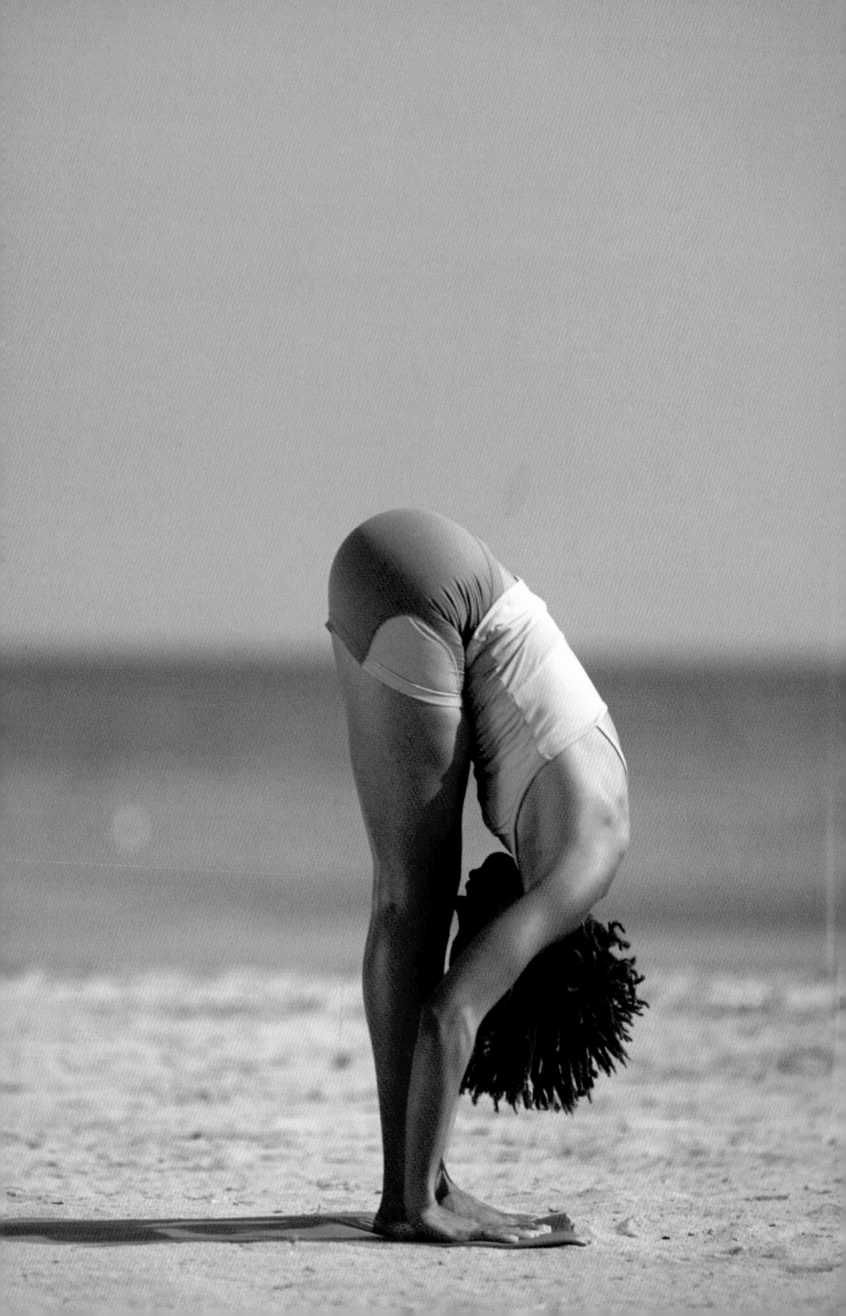

101

ESSENTIAL TIPS

Yoga

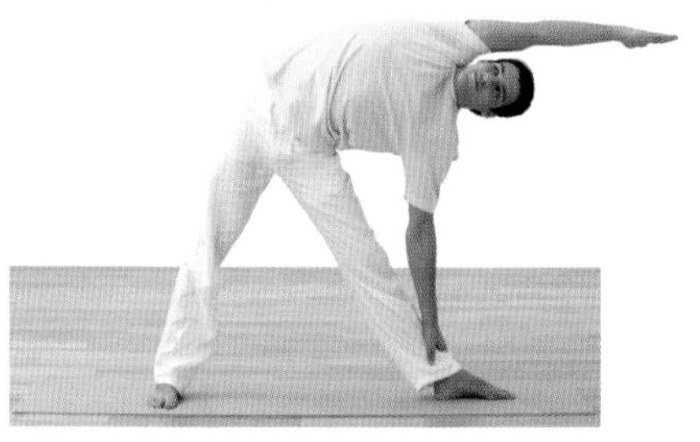

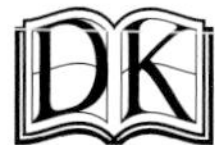

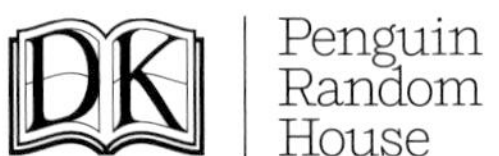

Produced for Dorling Kindersley by
Sands Publishing Solutions
4 Jenner Way, Eccles, Aylesford, Kent ME20 7SQ

Editorial Partners	David & Sylvia Tombesi-Walton
Design Partner	Simon Murrell
Project Editor	Chauney Dunford
Project Art Editor	Elaine Hewson
US Editor	Jill Hamilton
US Senior Editor	Shannon Beatty
Managing Editor	Penny Warren
Jacket Designer	Kathryn Wilding
Senior Pre-production Producer	Tony Phipps
Senior Producer	Ché Creasey
Art Director	Jane Bull
Publisher	Mary Ling
Consultant	Poggy Hatton

First American edition 2015
Published in the United States by
DK Publishing
345 Hudson Street, New York, New York 10014
A Penguin Random House Company

15 16 17 18 19 10 9 8 7 6 5 4 3 2 1

001-274503-May/2015

Published in Great Britain by Dorling Kindersley Limited.

A catalog record for this book is available from the Library of Congress.

ISBN 978-1-4654-2998-8

Printed and bound in China by South China Printing Co. Ltd.

A WORLD OF IDEAS:
SEE ALL THERE IS TO KNOW
www.dk.com

101 ESSENTIAL TIPS

Pages 8 to 19

YOGA & YOU

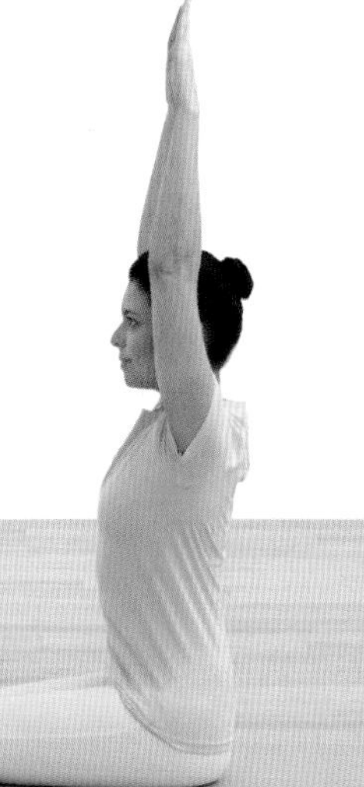

Pages 20 to 29

GETTING STARTED

Pages 30 to 43

POSES FOR STRENGTH

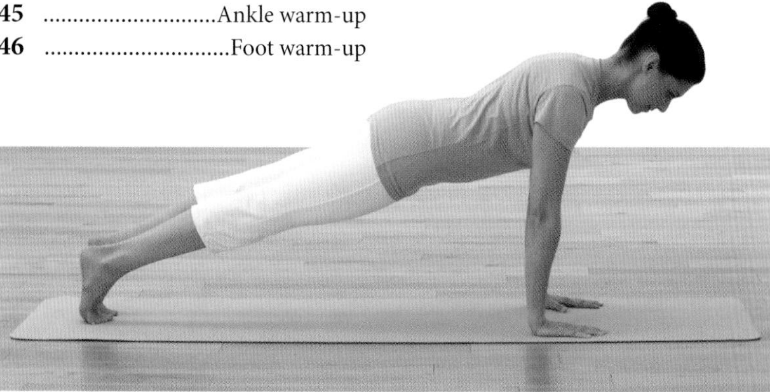

Pages 44 to 53

POSES FOR TONE & STRETCH

Pages 54 to 59

POSES FOR RELAXATION

Pages 60 to 63

POSES FOR BALANCE

Pages 64 to 69

THE COOL-DOWN

YOGA & YOU

1 WHAT IS YOGA?

The word "yoga" means "union." Yoga is a form of exercise based on the belief that the body and breath are intimately connected with the mind. By controlling the breath and holding the body in steady poses, or asanas, yoga creates harmony. Yoga consists of five key elements: beneficial exercise, correct breathing, complete relaxation, balanced diet, and positive thinking. The asanas help ease tension, tone internal organs, and improve flexibility.

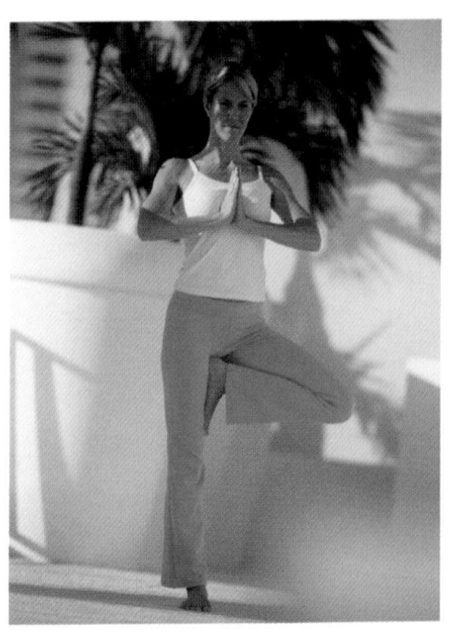

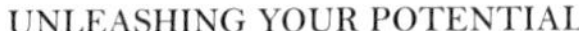

UNLEASHING YOUR POTENTIAL
Yoga helps create a flexible body coupled with a relaxed but focused mental state, able to tap into the full depths of its potential.

DIG DEEP
To maximize the benefits of yoga practice, hold postures steady for several breaths, reaching for a deeper stretch on each.

2 BENEFICIAL EXERCISE

The aim of yoga practice is to improve suppleness and strength. Each posture is performed slowly in fluid movements. Jerky movements should be avoided, because they produce a buildup of lactic acid, which causes fatigue. It is also important to take into account your existing fitness and stamina. Yoga postures can be modified to make them safe for people of all abilities.

Focus in on steady, rhythmic breathing
Feel expansion and contraction of abdomen

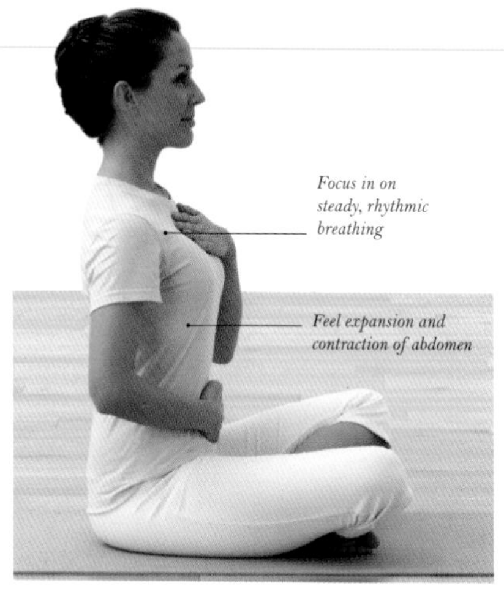

3 CORRECT BREATHING

Yogic breathing techniques maximize oxygen levels in your blood. Correct breathing is achieved through proper execution of the asanas, so be aware of the position of your chest, ensuring that you are connecting to the movement of the diaphragm. Deep exhalations also force stale air from the lungs, and breath control facilitates the calming of, and greater ability to focus, the mind.

4 COMPLETE RELAXATION

It is most beneficial to begin and end each yoga session with relaxation. You should also take a little time to relax between asanas. Relaxation sequences apply pressure to those areas of the body that are tense, massaging them in a similar way to acupressure to release the tension held there.

ABSOLUTE MINIMUM

The yoga definition of true relaxation is the point at which the body consumes the minimum amount of energy required to exist.

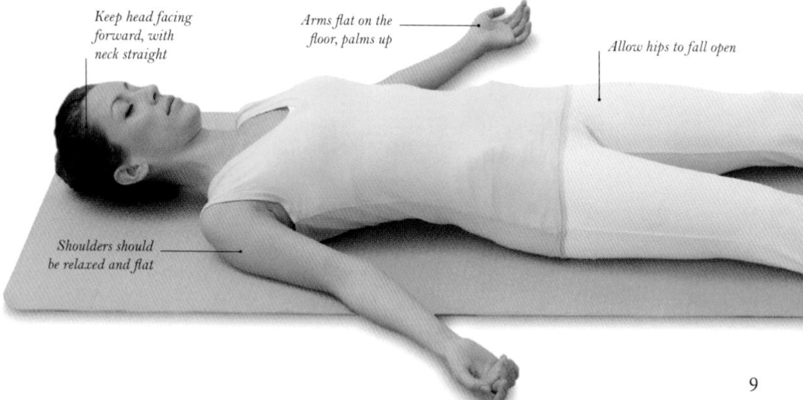

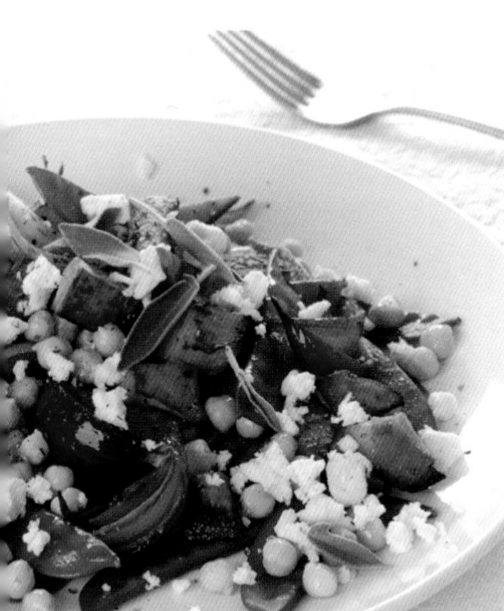

5 BALANCED DIET

The recommended yogic diet is very much in line with current ideas about healthy eating. It is a simple, wholesome vegetarian way of eating, comprised of natural foods that are easy to digest: fresh fruit and vegetables, dairy products, nuts, and legumes. It is also important to eat in moderation and only when hungry, taking time to chew food properly.

EATING HEALTHILY
As much as possible, make the healthy choice, by favoring natural fresh ingredients over processed and canned foods.

6 POSITIVE THINKING

In yoga, much importance is placed on the value of positive thinking in sustaining mental well-being. Through meditation and relaxation, yoga aims to clear the mind of negativity, while at the same time using positive affirmations to increase self-esteem. Some people think this is difficult to achieve, but practicing yoga will eventually bring you to a state of mental harmony and serenity.

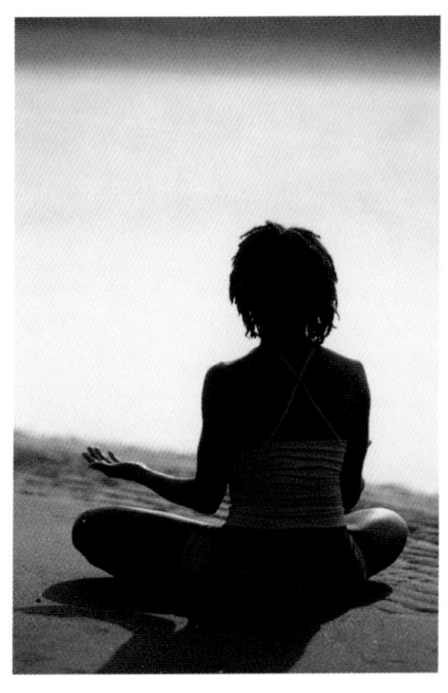

TAPPING INTO CREATIVITY
By channeling your thoughts in a positive direction, you will be better able to unlock your creative potential.

7 INCREASING VITALITY

Left unchecked, toxins build up in the body, leading to lethargy. Many yoga postures massage the internal organs that are involved in the elimination of waste products. This helps flush out toxins, thereby increasing vital nourishment to the organs and making your body function far more efficiently.

Palms pressed together, drawing upward
Lengthen through torso
Foot positioned as high as possible
Hold standing leg firm

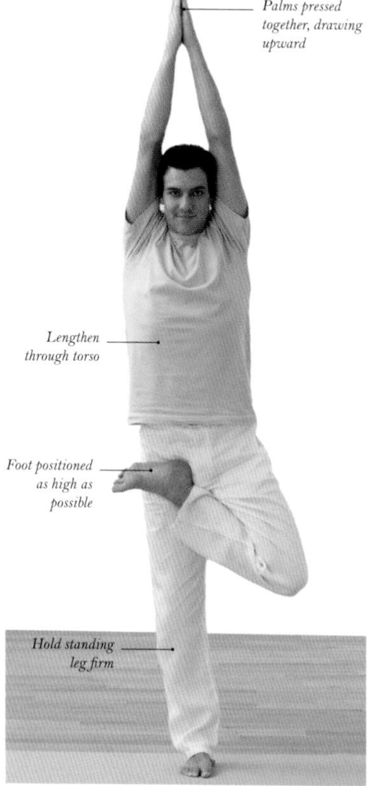

8 NURTURING THE NERVOUS SYSTEM

Practicing yoga can help the nervous system release blocked energy channels and activate healing. Postures that twist or bend the neck are particularly effective for putting the body into a restorative, healing mode. This state is also activated through the relaxation brought about by yogic breathing techniques.

Stretch up and back, with palms facing forward
Arch back, pushing chest forward
Inhale while stretching upward
Keep legs straight

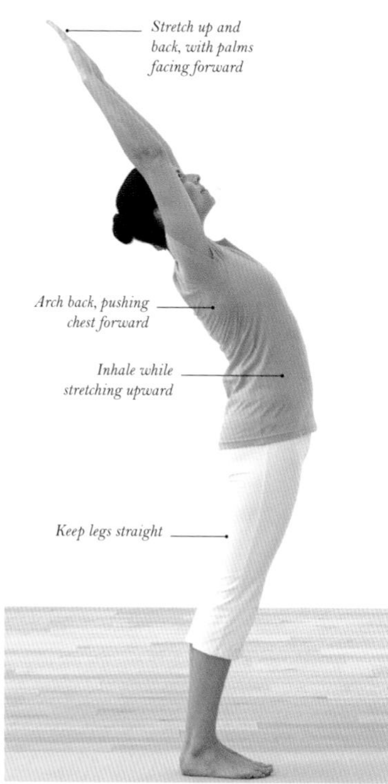

9 HEALTHY EATING

Consuming the right foods is an important part of bringing the mind and body into harmony. Foods that are beneficial to us are said to be Sattvic, or pure. Impure foods that can upset our physical, emotional, or intellectual balance are identified as being in the categories Tamasic (stale or rotten) and Rajasic (stimulating); foods that fall into these categories should be avoided by those following the yogic philosophy.

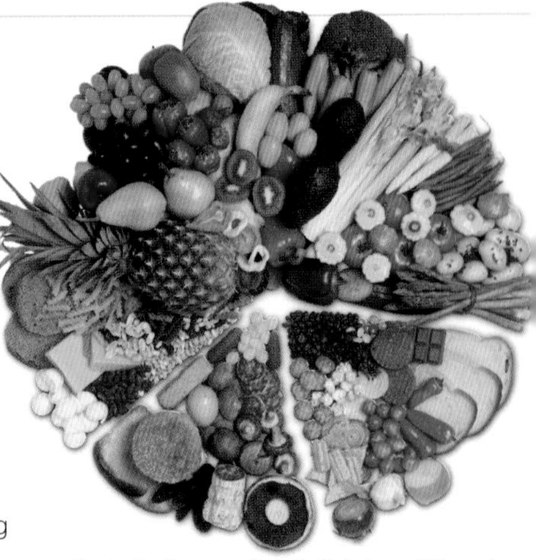

Clockwise from top: Sattvic, Rajasic, and Tamasic

FOODS TO EAT
Sattvic foods include the following: grains; fresh fruit and vegetables; natural fruit juices; dairy products such as milk, cheese, and butter; beans, nuts, and legumes; honey; and pure water.

FOODS TO AVOID
Tamasic foods include: meat and fish; mushrooms; and products that have been frozen, preserved, or canned. Rajasic items include: onions and garlic; tobacco; eggs; coffee and tea; strong spices; and chocolate.

10 AVOID ALCOHOL

Alcohol contains fermented products, introducing toxins into the body and overexciting the mind. Consequently, it is both Tamasic and Rajasic. Improve your mental clarity and physical well-being by avoiding alcohol.

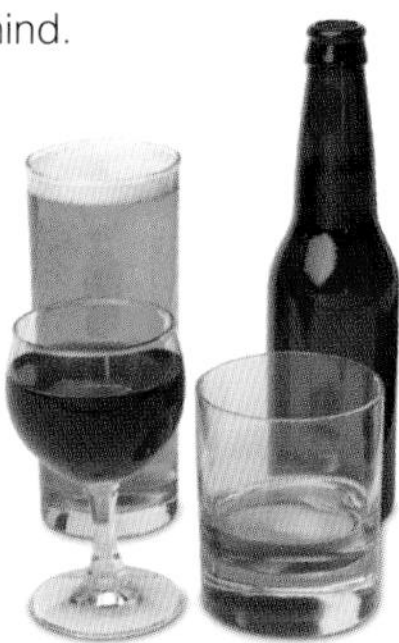

Remove all alcohol from your diet

11 DON'T SMOKE

Tobacco is another product that is both Rajasic and Tamasic. By giving up smoking you will eliminate toxins from your body, helping you achieve a calm mind and body.

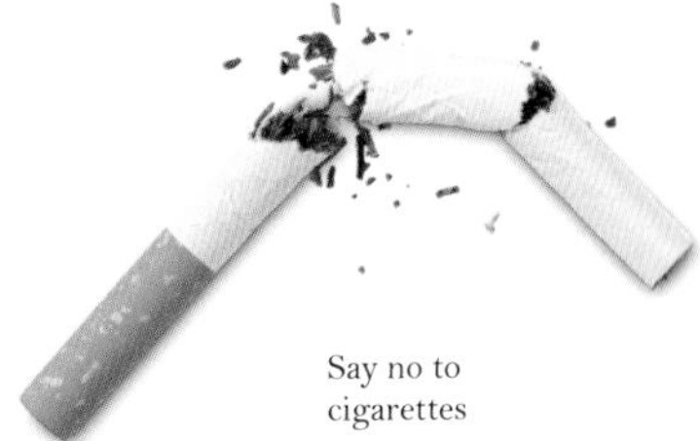

Say no to cigarettes

12 CARE FOR YOUR BACK

Yoga postures flex and extend each section of the spine to help it regain its inherent flexibility. Each of the vertebrae goes through the full range of movement in all directions, although to varying degrees depending on the pose. The increased mobility of the intervertebral disks reduces injuries, since there is less strain on movement. The postures work on toning and strengthening the muscles that support the back, giving additional support to the spine.

Turn head to right
Press elbow against knee

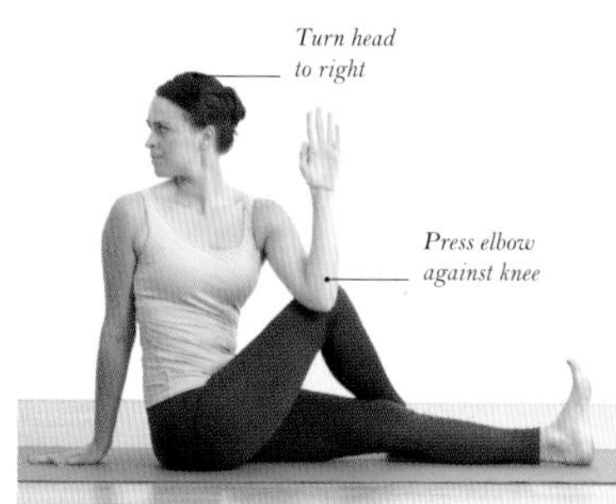

HALF SPINAL TWIST
The benefits of this pose (see p.39) include strengthening of the back and thighs, as well as improving your posture.

Rotate head to left
Bring left thigh over right leg
Keep left foot relaxed

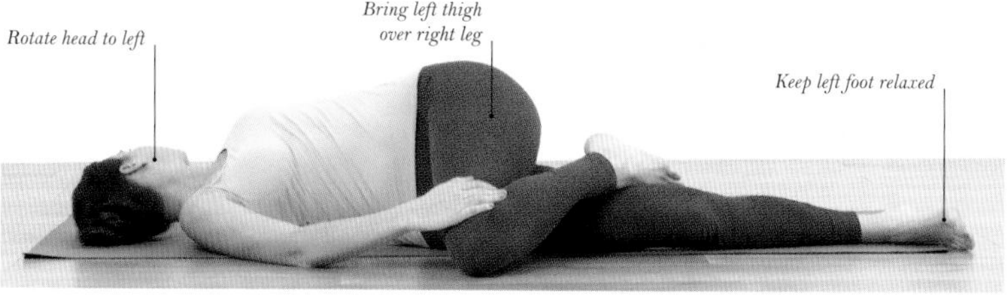

EASY FLOOR TWIST
This posture (see p.57) helps relieve tension in the back. The twisting motion helps in the revitalization of the abdominal organs.

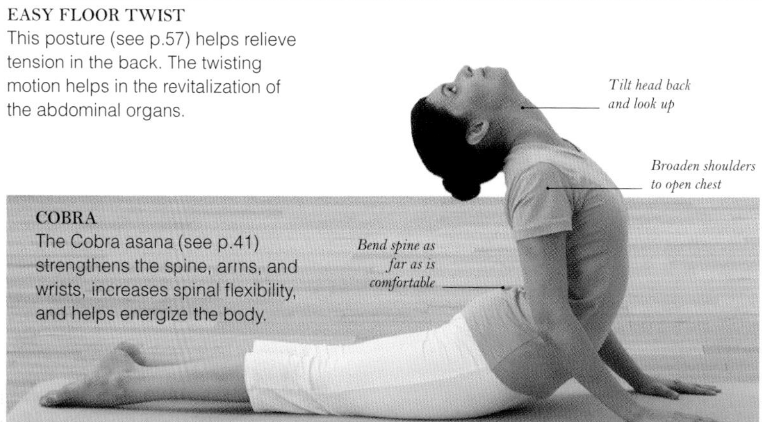

COBRA
The Cobra asana (see p.41) strengthens the spine, arms, and wrists, increases spinal flexibility, and helps energize the body.

13 ENERGIZE YOUR SPINE

Yoga asanas flex and extend different sections of the spine to varying degrees in order to develop spinal flexibility. The poses that offer the most obvious benefits for the spine include back and forward bends and twists. Such postures help maintain and restore the spine's support network, such as the ligaments that bind vertebrae together, spinal joints, and the disks between the vertebrae, as well as the surrounding muscles.

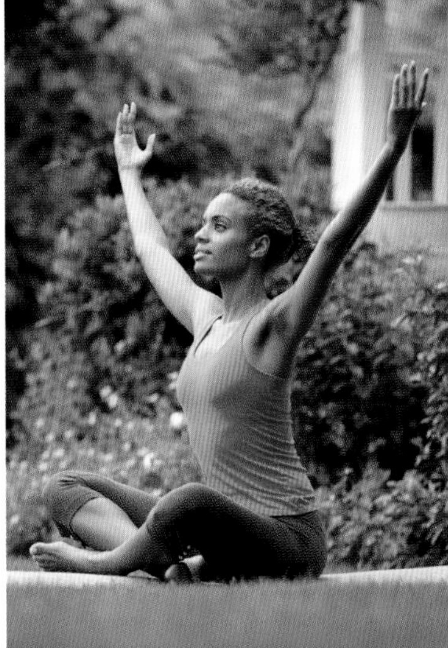

CORRECTING CURVATURE
Yoga poses help correct any abnormal curvatures of the spine that may have developed through poor posture.

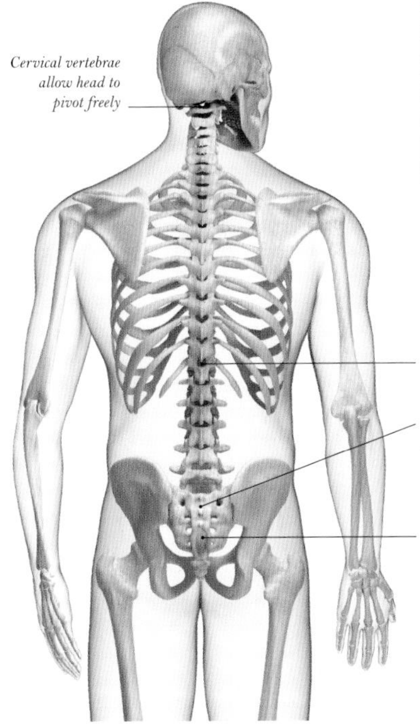

NOURISHING THE SPINAL CORD
A flexible spine nourishes the cerebrospinal fluid that surrounds the spinal cord and allows *prana*, or vital energy, to flow freely throughout the body.

14 ALIGNING YOUR BODY

The cornerstone of yoga is learning to hold your body in line. Consider the body as a single unit that is segmented into eight parts—head, torso, arms, forearms, hands, thighs, legs, and feet—and remember that the straight line can be horizontal, vertical, or angled, depending on the particular yoga posture you are attempting.

INTERNAL MIRROR

Try to create a mind-map, or "internal mirror," of your body. Use this to realign the body by working slowly up, from the toes to the head. Make tiny adjustments until you feel grounded and centered. Become aware of your breathing pattern as you ease into correct alignment.

Raise arms straight up, palms facing inward
Tilt head back slightly
Inhale as you lift arms

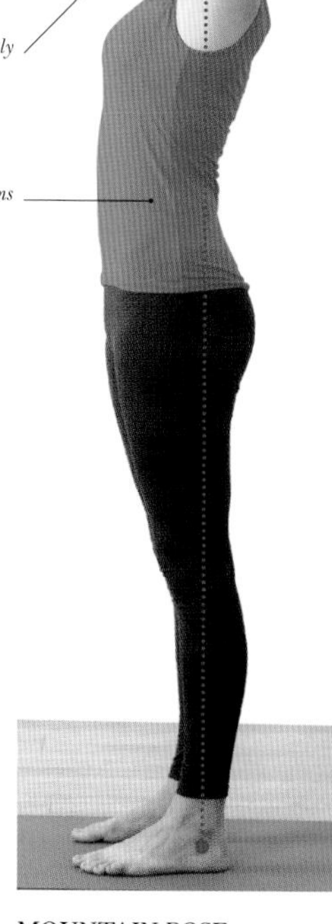

MOUNTAIN POSE
This yoga exercise (see p.30) is perfect for helping achieve spinal alignment, as well as for improving your posture.

15 BALANCE BOTH SIDES

In everyday life, many activities work or emphasize one part or side of the body. However, for balance and harmony, it is important to keep all body parts equally strong. That is why in yoga the same exercises are repeated on both sides of the body.

Stretch as far as possible on one side
Stretch to the same extent on the other side

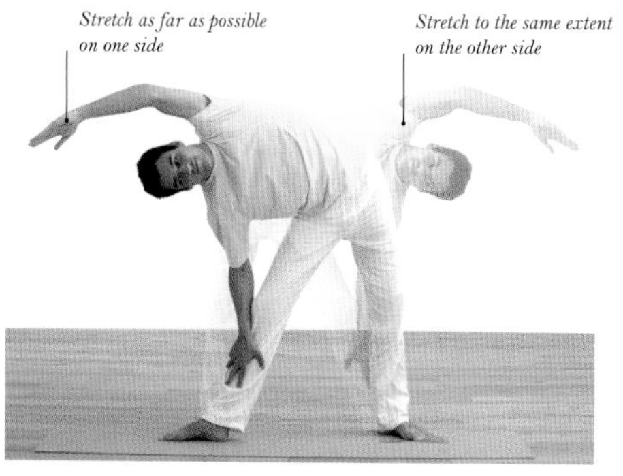

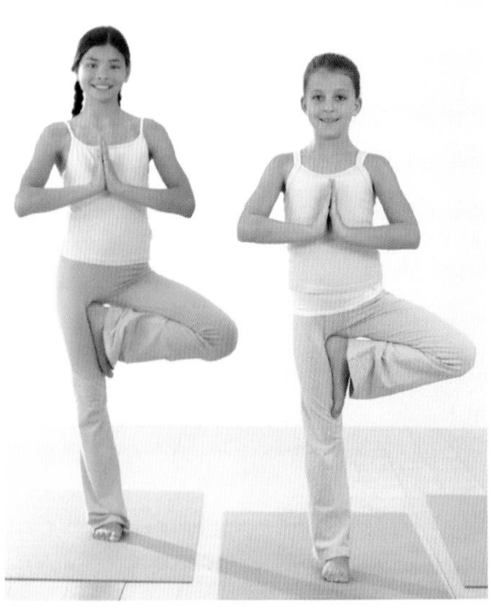

YOGA FOR THE YOUNG

For children, yoga is a great way to develop self-awareness, self-control, and powers of concentration. If you have kids, encourage them to join you in your yoga practice. They are likely to be flexible even if they lack stamina. However, the latter will increase with regular sessions.

COPYCAT KIDS

Children have a natural curiosity and desire to mimic, so they will probably be intrigued enough by your yoga to want to join in.

YOGA FOR THE PREGNANT

Practicing yoga during the prenatal period can be a valuable learning experience. Also, it can help ease your pregnancy, as well as the delivery. Work slowly and gently, allowing the poses to relax and strengthen the body and to help it adjust to the changes that are happening within. However, talk to your instructor about which poses should not be attempted while pregnant.

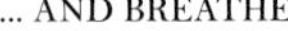

... AND BREATHE

Yogic breathing exercises—always important—come into their own during pregnancy, helping you make the most of your breath.

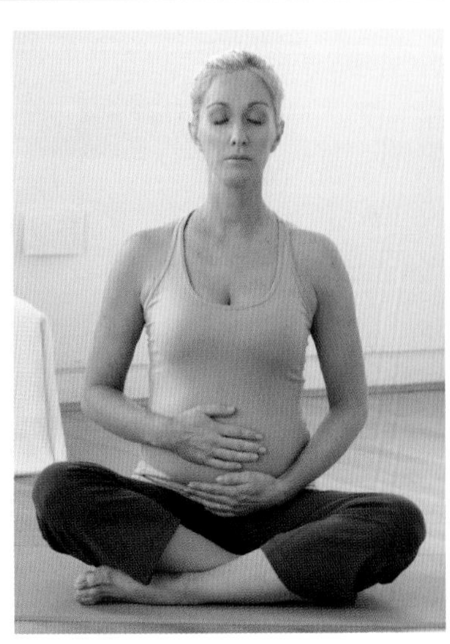

18 YOGA FOR THE ELDERLY

There is no age limit for yoga, in part because it is noncompetitive and you work at your own pace. Done correctly, there is no risk of injury, and regular practice helps maintain good health and mobility. Additionally, yoga stimulates circulation and reduces the effects of arthritis.

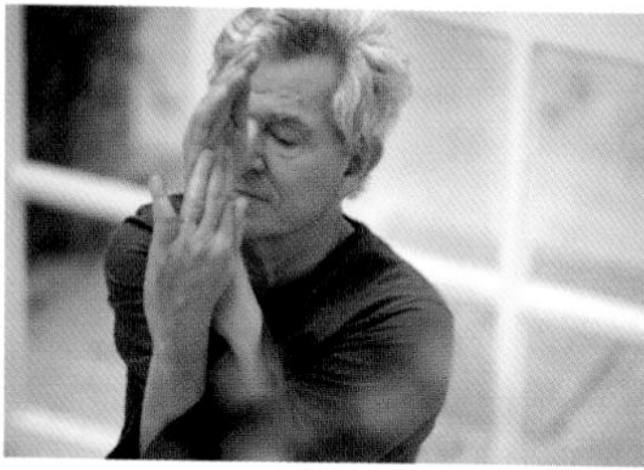

Don't let advancing years deter you

19 YOGA FOR STRESS

Many yoga asanas help relieve stress by releasing tension that has built up in your body. Breathing exercises and meditation are also helpful, since they relax the body and calm the mind. Mental tranquillity can be further encouraged by avoiding stimulants.

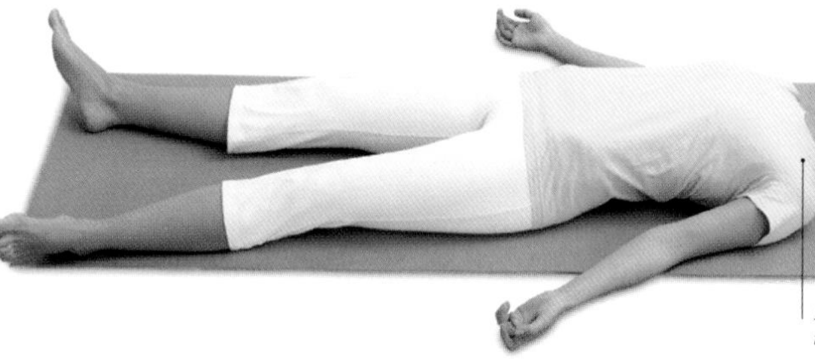

Calm the mind with breathing and meditation

Ease tension by relaxing the body fully

20 YOGA FOR RELAXATION

Just as relaxing the body and mind helps get you ready for your yoga practice, your regular sessions make it easier for you to maintain a relaxed state in general—and easier to achieve that relaxed state when you are feeling the stresses and strains of daily life. The warm-up exercises on pp.26–29 are a great start, but see also the poses in Chapter 5, as well as the cool-down relaxation on pp.64–65.

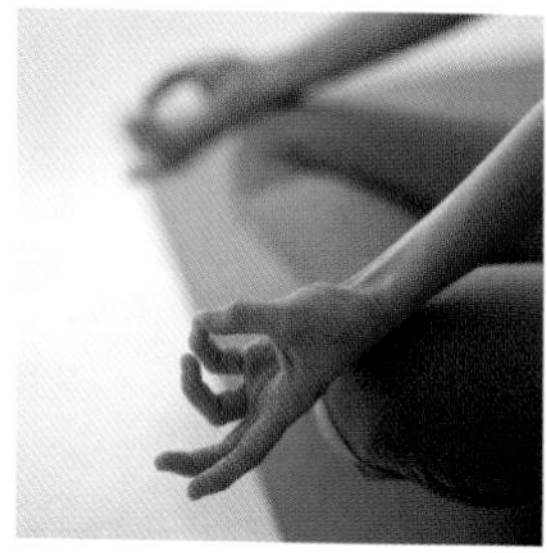

Yoga helps you connect to yourself

21 WHEN TO PRACTICE YOGA

Because yoga ought to be practiced on an empty stomach, early mornings or evenings tend to be the best times, but you need to consider what suits you best. Morning practice awakens the body and eases stiffness by lubricating the joints and energizing the muscles. Digestion is stimulated and mental alertness is increased, ready for a productive day. Conversely, evening yoga can help counter the stresses of the day, improving the quality of your sleep. Whichever you choose, setting aside a regular time is good for establishing a routine.

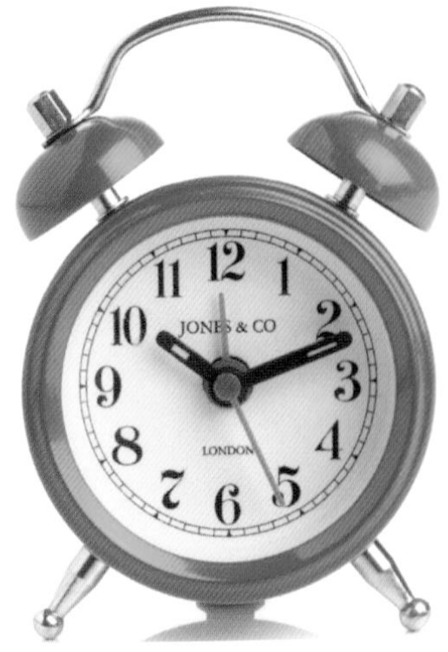

22 WHERE TO PRACTICE YOGA

You don't need a special room or fancy equipment for yoga, but there are some things to consider when choosing a practice place. Ideally, opt for a private area away from distractions. If that area is spacious, even better, since this can have a positive effect on the mind and, therefore, help you relax. Try to personalize the space, too, because this can also calm the mind.

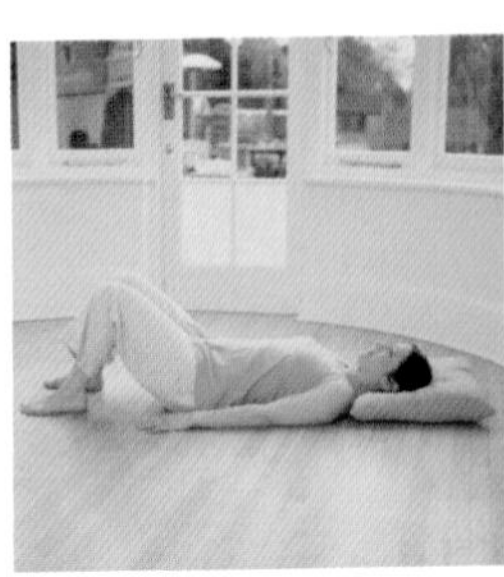

LIGHT AND AIRY
Ideally your space ought to be lit by natural light and have some form of ventilation. The floor should be level, firm, and nonslip.

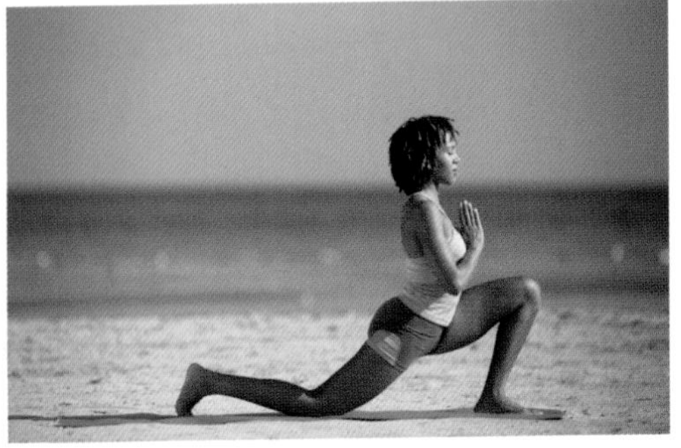

OPEN-AIR YOGA
If you are lucky enough to be near a quiet, flat open space, take advantage of it. Lay down your mat, and greet the day with open-air yoga.

23 YOGA CLASSES

Regardless of how small or large your class, it is always best to have your yoga practice supervised by a qualified teacher at least until you are confident. This is the only way to learn how to ease your body correctly into and out of the asanas, as well as how to breathe correctly when holding a pose. Your teacher will also make sure you do not strain your limbs.

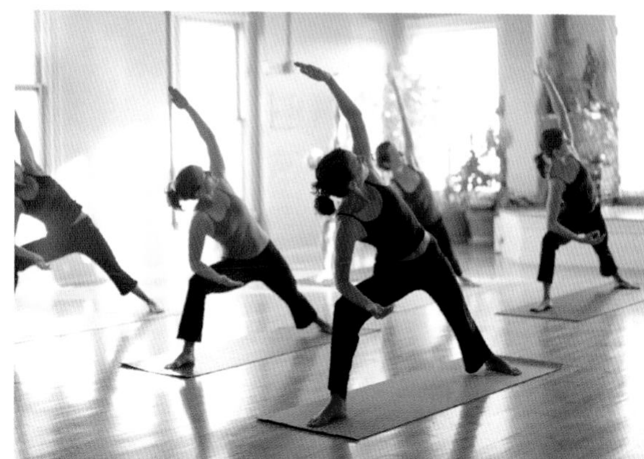

EXPERT HELP
Get your yoga practice off to the best possible start by taking classes. They will also help you improve your technique and build your confidence.

24 YOGA AT HOME

Yoga's portability means that, once you have some experience, you will be able to practice the postures in the comfort of your own home. Indeed, your teacher may even suggest that you work at home with some of the simpler asanas or with the relaxation techniques.

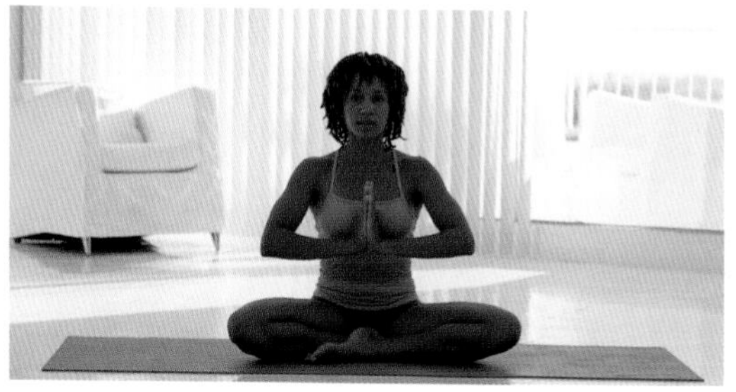

MINIMAL REQUIREMENTS
With just yourself and a mat (or a comfortable floor), it is perfectly possible to practice yoga at home.

GETTING STARTED

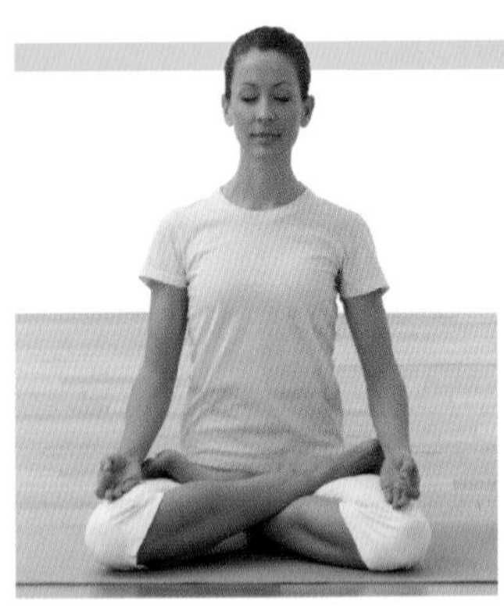

25 KNOW YOUR BODY

Before you undertake any yoga practice, first take the time to understand your body, bearing in mind any factors that might affect its performance, such as recent surgery, pregnancy, or medical conditions.

CHECK FOR TENSION

While in an asana, check for any tension and try to relax it with your breathing.

26 UNDERSTAND YOUR LIMITS

It is important to know what your body's limits are and not to force yourself to go beyond them. There is no rush; yoga is completely noncompetitive. Continue your regular yoga sessions and you will find your body becomes more flexible with time.

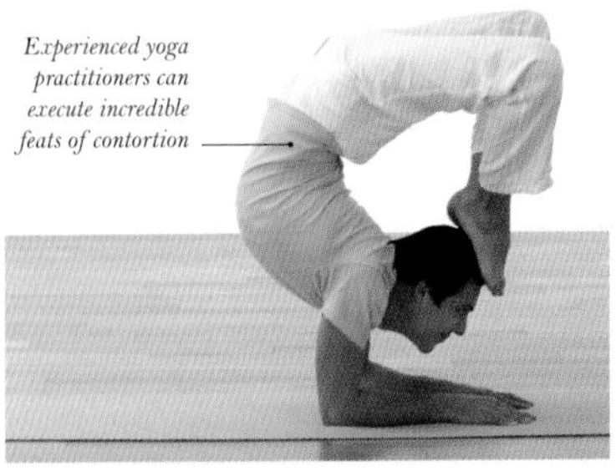

Experienced yoga practitioners can execute incredible feats of contortion

27 CONSULT A DOCTOR

Regardless of age, yoga is perfectly appropriate for everyone. Nevertheless, as with any physical exercise, if you have any medical concerns or conditions, it is a good idea to check with your doctor before beginning a class.

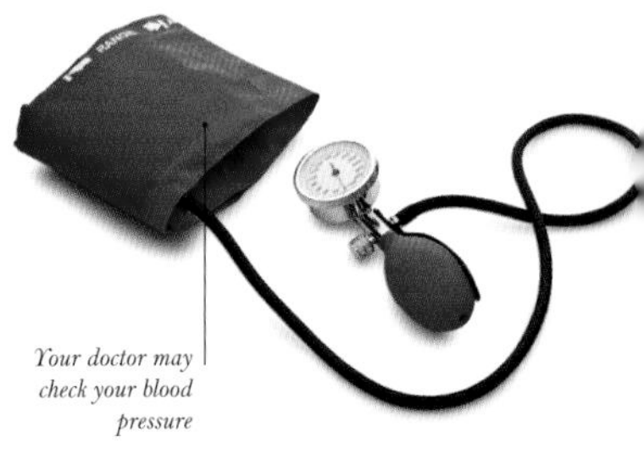

Your doctor may check your blood pressure

28 ESSENTIAL EQUIPMENT

Yoga equipment will keep you safer and more comfortable while you practice. Some pieces, such as blocks and straps, can also be used to help you achieve poses that would otherwise be beyond your capabilities, as you continue to work on expanding your level of flexibility. Props and supports can also extend the time you can hold a pose with proper body alignment.

YOGA KIT CHECKLIST

The equipment you are most likely to need or find useful in your yoga practice comprises:

- Slip-resistant mat
- Block, usually foam
- Strap or belt
- Cushion
- Towel

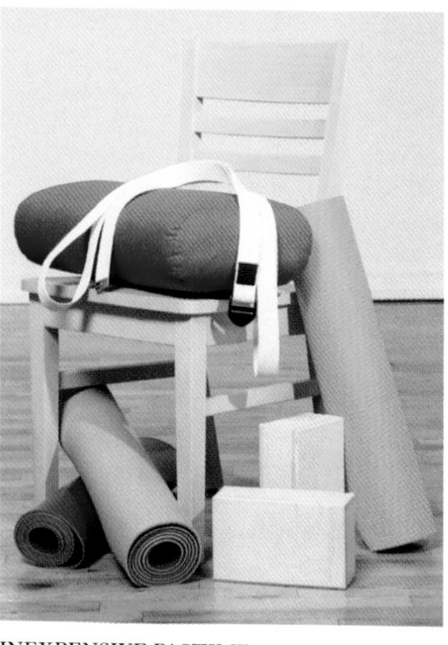

INEXPENSIVE PASTIME

Most yoga teachers will have equipment for use in classes, but it is all affordable enough to make it worth investing in your own.

29 WHAT TO WEAR

Whatever you wear for your yoga sessions should be comfortable and must allow complete freedom of movement. Ideally, you would practice in bare feet, but socks are fine. If practical to do so, also remove any dangling jewelry before beginning your session because it may distract or annoy you.

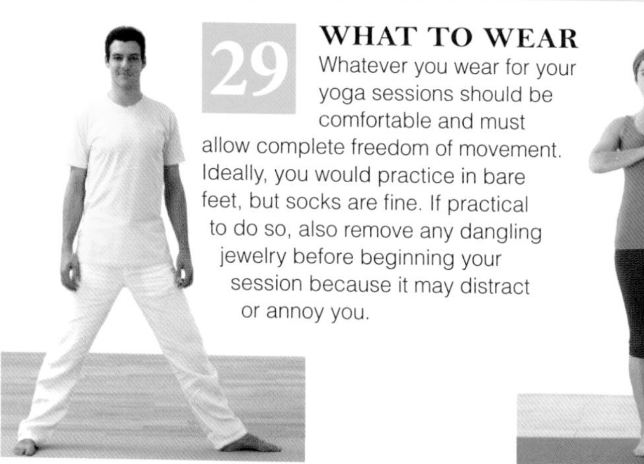

Lightweight, loose-fitting clothes

Tight, stretch-material clothes

30 PLAN YOUR SESSIONS

More experienced yoga practitioners working alone may find it useful to create a plan in advance of each session, or to work out the sequence of asanas. This will save time because you don't have to choose between postures during the session.

SAMPLE WORKOUT

1. Mountain Pose
2. Triangle Pose
3. Warrior 2
4. Extended Side Stretch
5. Downward-Facing Dog
6. Warrior
7. Warrior Lunge
8. Cobra
9. Cat Balance
10. Plank
11. Child's Pose
12. Cobbler
13. Corpse Pose

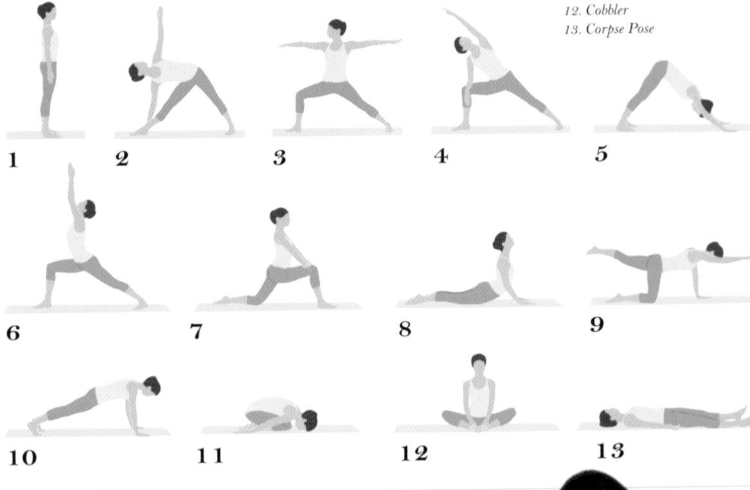

31 KEEP A YOGA JOURNAL

Writing in a yoga journal after each session will help you track your goals and accomplishments, as well as allowing you to identify any problem areas that need more attention. A yoga journal can also act as a means of reinforcing your practice so you can more easily tailor it to your own needs.

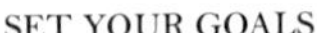

SET YOUR GOALS

Although yoga is not a competitive pursuit, it can be fun and rewarding to set your own goals in a yoga journal.

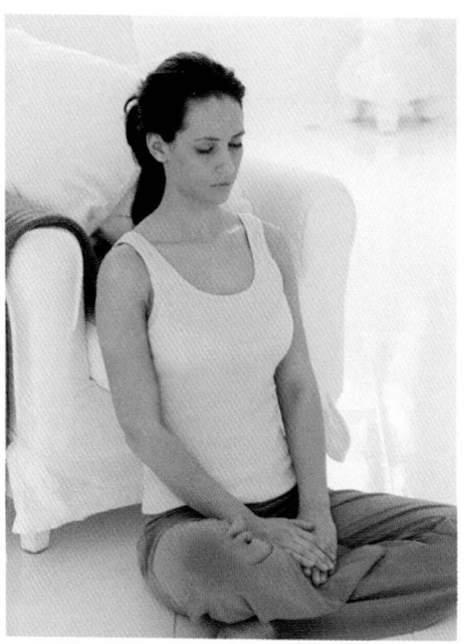

32 MONITOR YOUR PROGRESS

It's important when practicing any discipline to have a way of tracking progress. As well as keeping a yoga journal, a good method of self-assessment is to listen to your body. This requires practice and concentration, but once you are attuned to your body, you will be able to identify the benefits of your practice.

REFLECT FOR A MOMENT

Take time to reflect on your progress. This will help you build a firm foundation for your future yoga sessions.

33 SIMPLIFY POSES

When you first start yoga, you will almost certainly experience some stiffness and soreness in the joints. This shows you are working areas that may have been neglected. Building flexibility in these parts requires patience and commitment. If you find a specific pose hard, practice a modified version until you can progress.

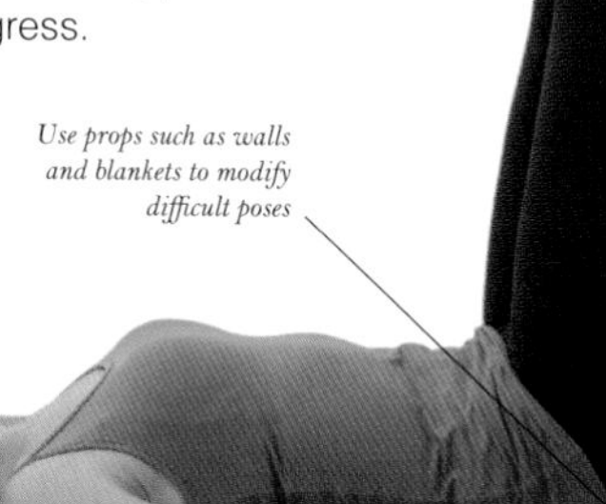

Use props such as walls and blankets to modify difficult poses

34 USING PROPS FOR STANDING POSITIONS

Forward bends and other standing postures may be beyond your reach to perform correctly when you first attempt them. Blocks or other means of support—a chair, for example—can be used to modify the posture so that increased flexibility can be gradually attained without injuring yourself.

Keep back straight and in line with arms
Keep feet hip-width apart
Chair should be high enough to achieve straight line from tailbone to hands

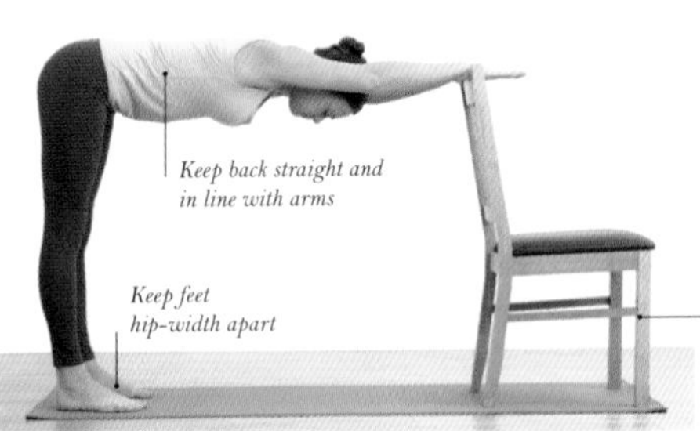

Using a chair for additional support

Using a block to support the head

35 USING PROPS FOR FLOOR POSES

By using a strap or a belt, you can start working toward achieving a posture that would otherwise be impossible for you when you first begin to practice yoga. When lying down, cushions and blankets can help provide the comfort you need in order to relax fully.

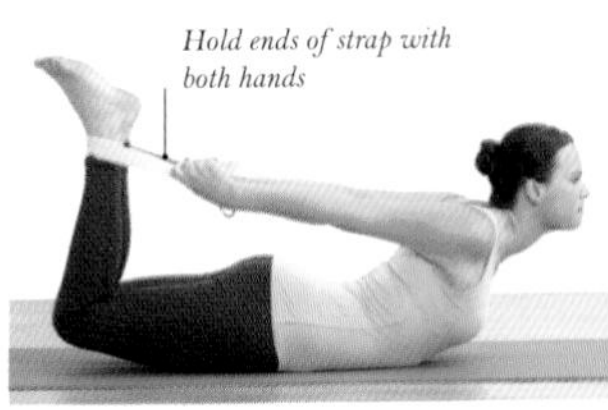

Hold ends of strap with both hands

Using a strap

Supports can be used to reduce discomfort

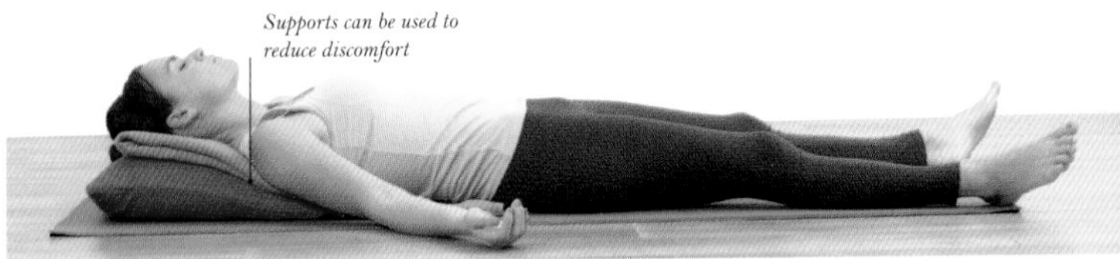

Using a cushion and a folded blanket

36 ABDOMINAL BREATHING

It is important to learn how to breathe efficiently for yoga. Lying on your back, place your hands on either side of your navel. Feel how the abdomen expands as you inhale and contracts as you exhale. By breathing slowly and deeply, you are able to take air into the lowest parts of your lungs, while also exercising your diaphragm.

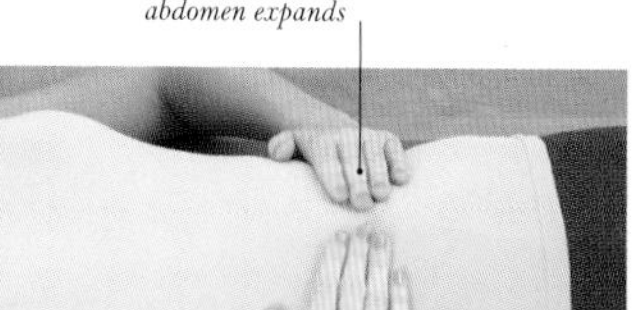

Inhalation

Fingers touch as abdomen contracts

Exhalation

37 HOW TO INHALE & EXHALE

Inhalation can be used to lengthen and expand within an asana, while exhalation helps release deeper into the pose. Careful and progressive work within postures will allow for a full, easy-flowing breath, which is a crucial indicator of how well the asana is being executed. In this respect, the breath and asana practice must work together.

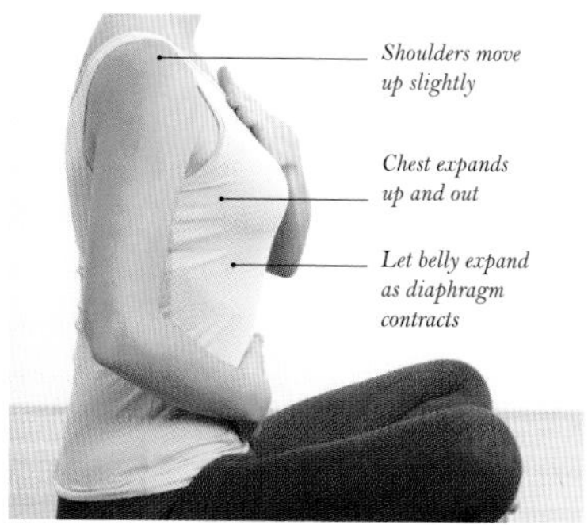

Inhalation

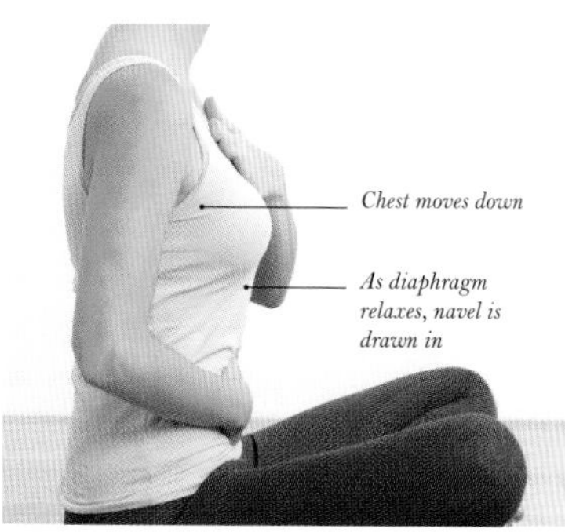

Exhalation

38 THE IMPORTANCE OF WARMING UP

Before beginning a yoga session, make sure you are fully warmed up. Carry out the exercises shown in Tips 39–46. You should also take some time to practice your breathing techniques (see Tips 36 and 37). Mastering breath control will allow you to breathe more deeply, enable you to position yourself correctly in the yoga asanas, and assist you in holding the poses.

39 EYE WARM-UP

This series of exercises is purely for the eyes, so be sure not to move the head or neck while doing them. Look up (below left). Look right (below middle left). Look up diagonally to the right (middle right). Look down (right). Repeat the sequence, this time looking to the left side and up diagonally to the left. Hold each position for a few seconds.

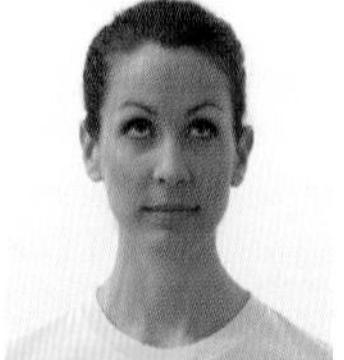

Looking up

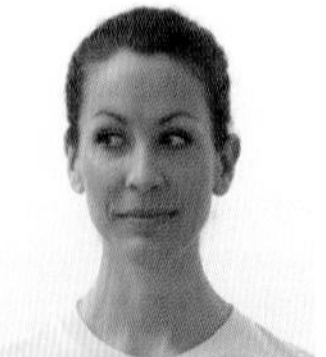

Looking right

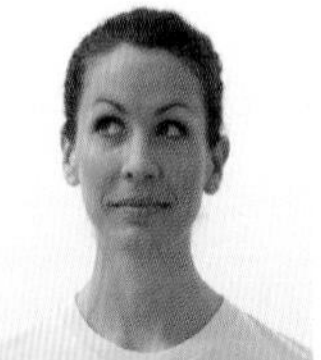

Looking up and right

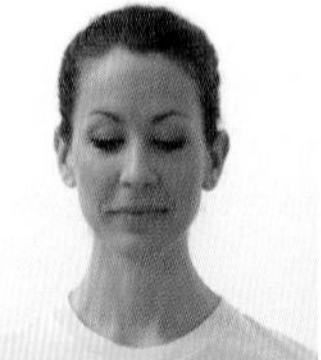

Looking down

40 NECK WARM-UP

Sit upright with your back straight. Slowly tilt your head forward, and then backward. Then tilt your head to the right, before repeating the same to the left. Finally, rotate your head 90 degrees to the right and then again to the left side. Hold each position for a few seconds. Never move your neck beyond what is comfortable.

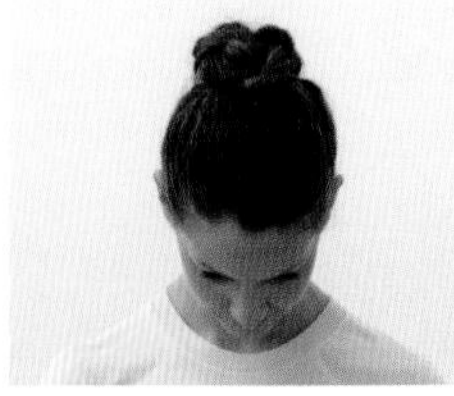

Tilting head forward

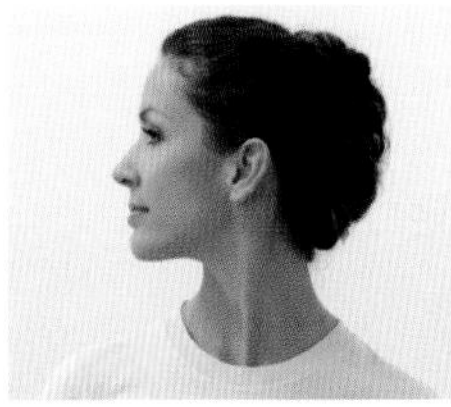

Rotating head to the right

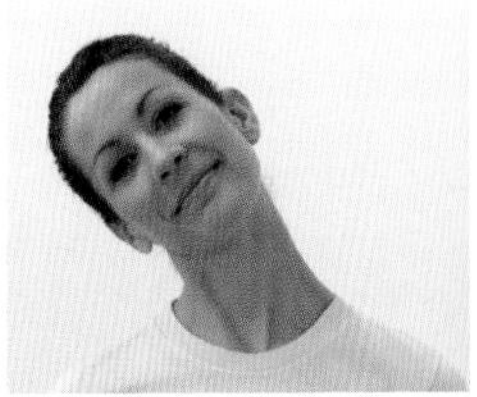

Tilting head to the right

41 SHOULDER WARM-UP

Stand upright with your fingertips on your shoulders and your elbows out to the side. Inhale, bringing your elbows in front of you so they touch. Exhale, lifting the elbows up and apart, stretching them up. Finally, lower the elbows down. Repeat ten times.

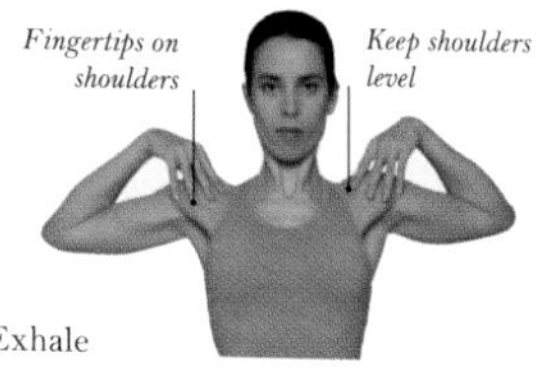

Exhale

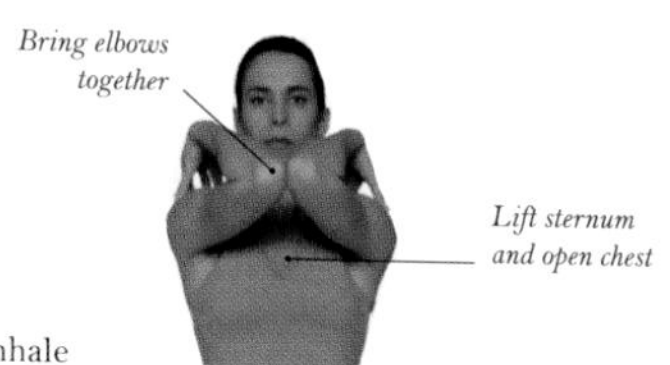

Inhale

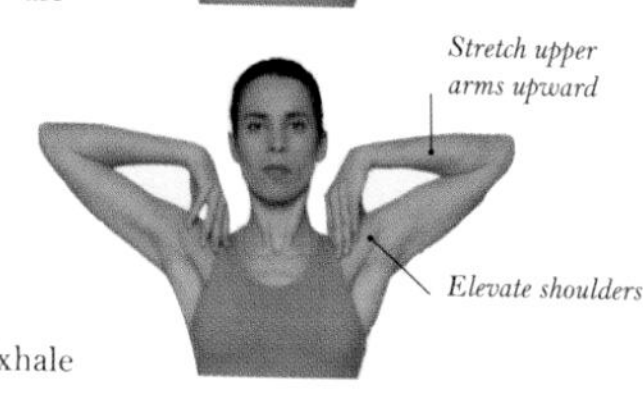

Exhale

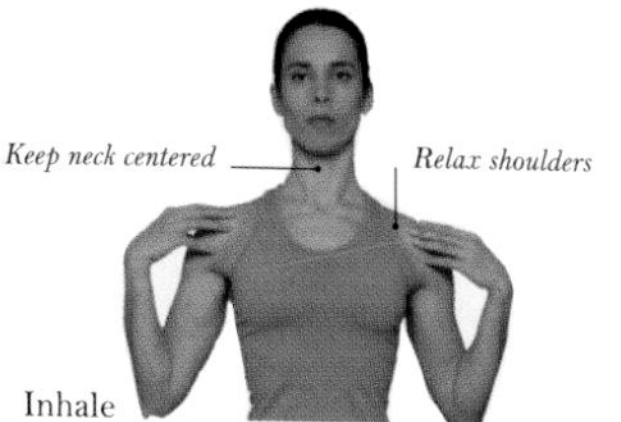

Inhale

42 TORSO WARM-UP

Start by standing with your feet hip-width apart and your palms resting on your hips. Gently and rhythmically, twist your upper body side to side, rotating at the hips, waist, and spine. Perform ten twists on each side, also allowing your head and shoulders to go with the movement.

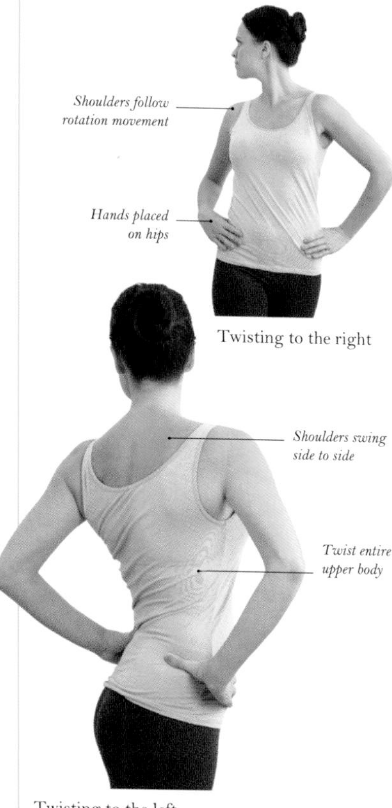

Twisting to the right

Twisting to the left

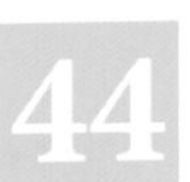

43 HIP WARM-UP

Start by standing with your feet hip-width apart, and put your hands on your hips. Keeping your legs straight and kneecaps pulled up, rotate the hips in a circle, ten times clockwise and ten times counterclockwise. Make sure you engage the hips and upper body in the roll.

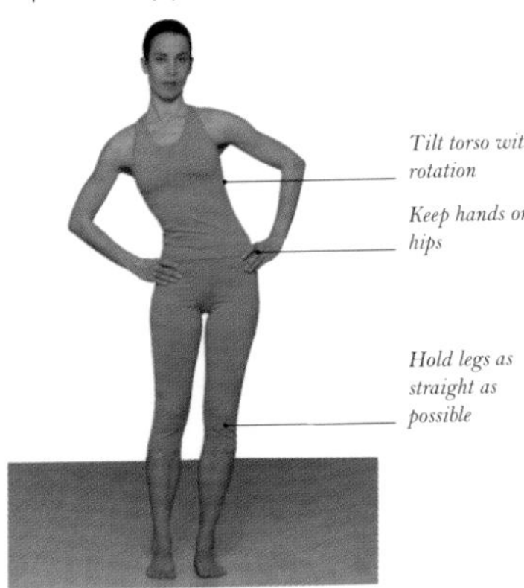

Rotating the hips clockwise

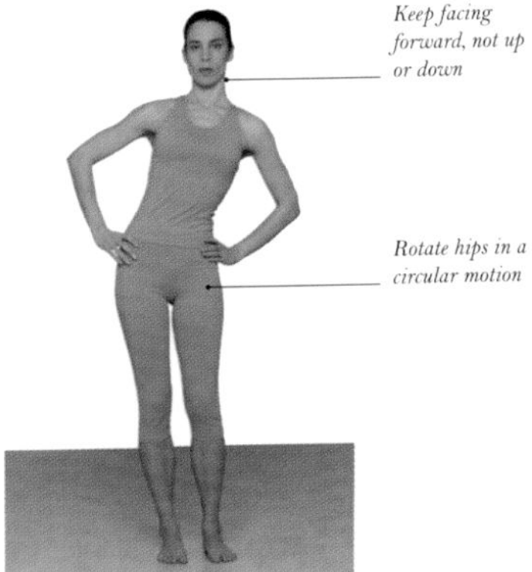

Rotating the hips counterclockwise

44 KNEE WARM-UP

Stand with your feet together and with your legs slightly bent at the knees. Bring your hands to rest lightly on your kneecaps, with fingers pointing downward. Rotate your knees gently in a circular motion, ten times in each direction, keeping your feet firmly rooted to the ground.

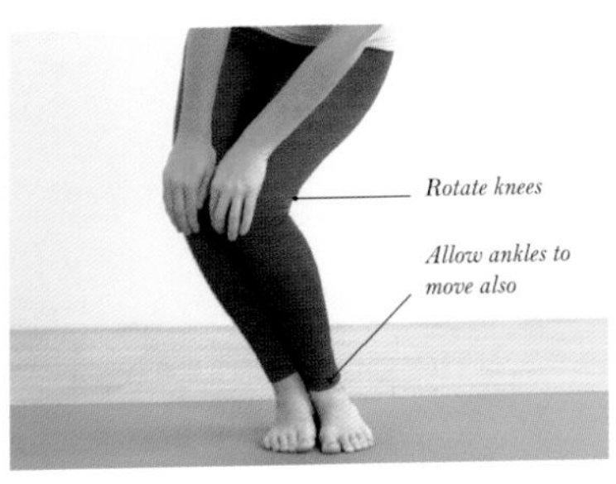

Rotating the knees clockwise

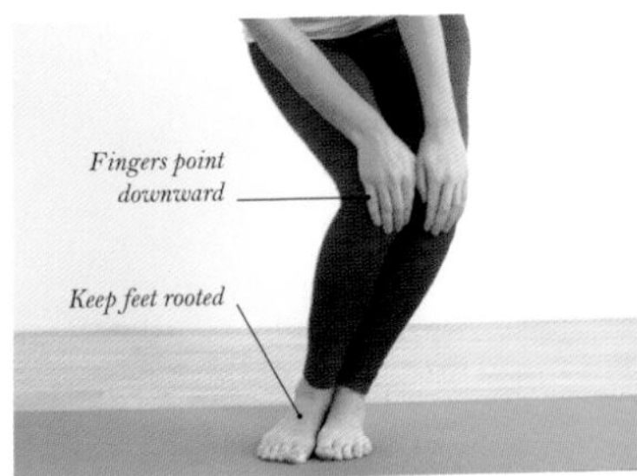

Rotating the knees counterclockwise

45 ANKLE WARM-UP

From a standing position, lift your right leg slightly, keeping the left leg firm. Balance yourself, then gently swing the right leg, toes pointing down. Hold for a few breaths before switching legs. Follow this by gently rotating the right foot at the ankle—first one way, then the other. Repeat with the left foot.

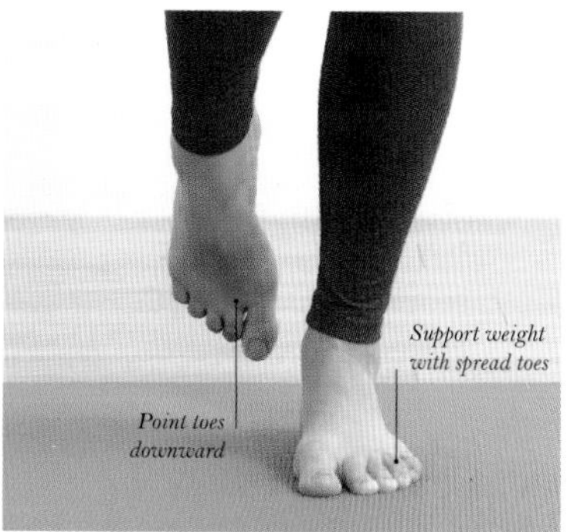

Leg swinging, with toes pointing down

Rotating the right ankle

FOOT WARM-UP

The feet should be stretched in both directions. First, stretch the heels a few times. Do this by lifting the right heel up as far as possible, then lowering it. Next, roll onto the front of the right toes, curling and gently pressing them under the foot. Hold for 2–3 breaths, then repeat on the left.

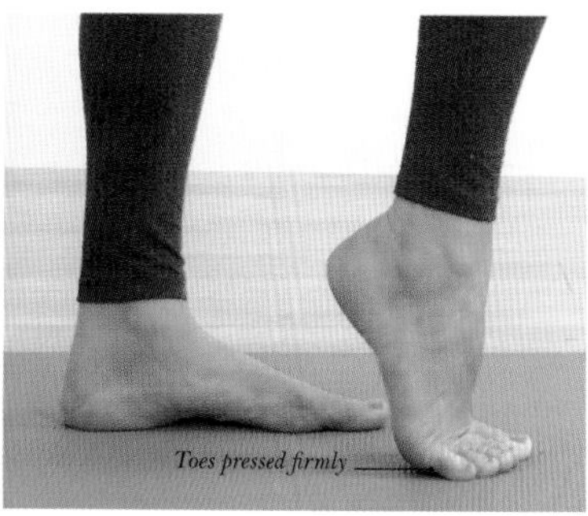

Stretching the heel

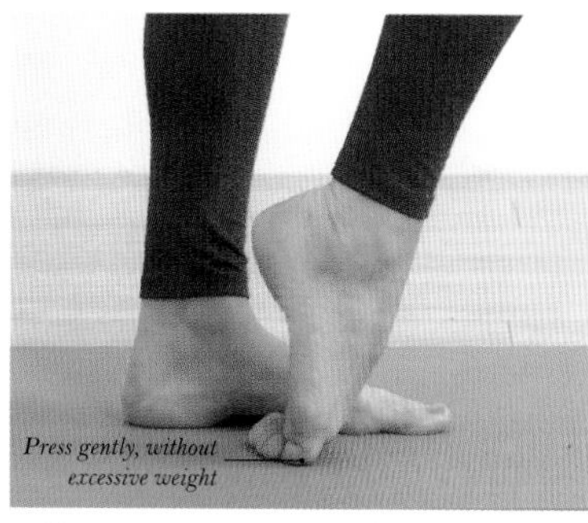

Rolling on to the toes

POSES FOR STRENGTH

47 HOW YOGA IMPROVES STRENGTH

All yoga asanas improve overall strength by engaging the core muscles, as well as other muscle groups depending on the pose. The muscles work to maintain balance and poise, getting stronger by moving through a range of motions while supporting the body's weight. The key to building strength over time is consistent yoga practice. Cardiovascular strength can be enhanced by regularly including the Sun Salutation (see Tip 62) in your practice, increasing both your heart rate and blood flow.

48 MOUNTAIN POSE

This posture is perfect for helping you correct spinal alignment. Start with your arms by your sides, feet hip-width apart, the sides of the legs parallel, and the toes pointing forward and pressed into the ground.

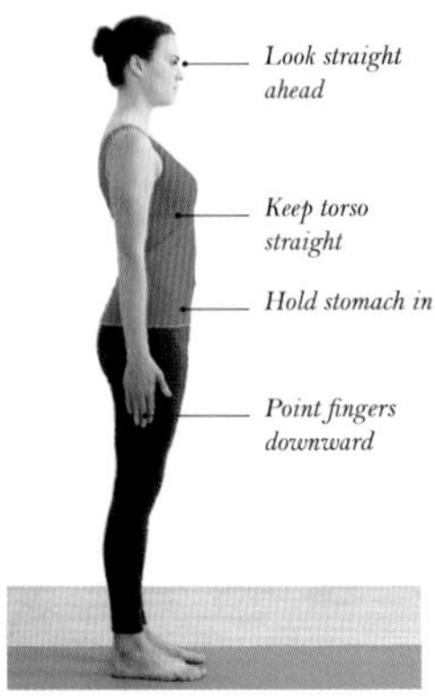

1 Realign your body slowly, from toes to head via ankles, knees, pelvis, chest, shoulders, and neck.

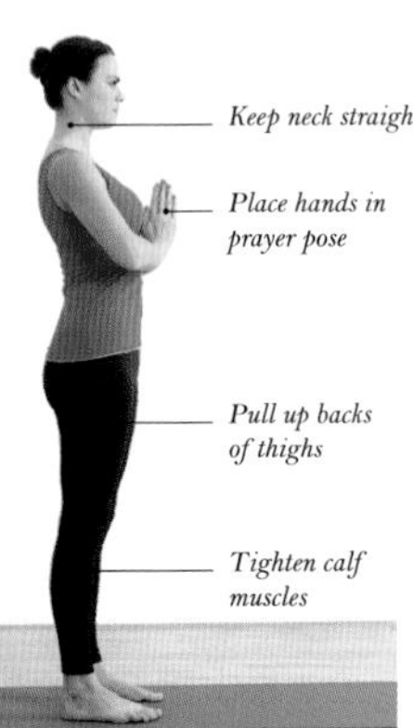

2 Bring your hands in front of your chest in prayer pose. Be sure to keep your head and neck straight.

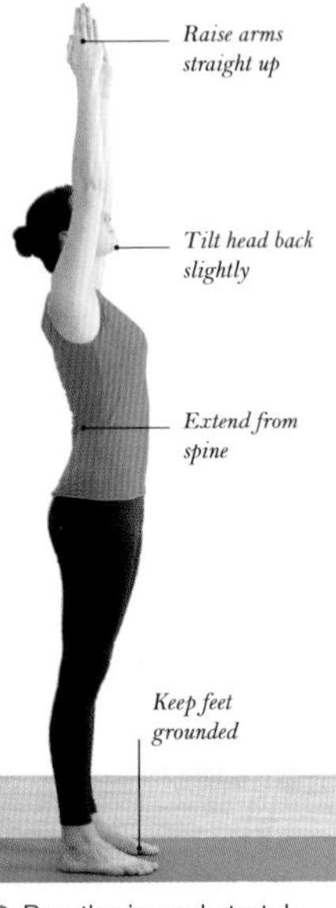

3 Breathe in and stretch the arms up, palms in, and tilt the neck up slightly. Lengthen the spine.

Release tension
in shoulders
Keep spine
straight
Position palms
on thighs

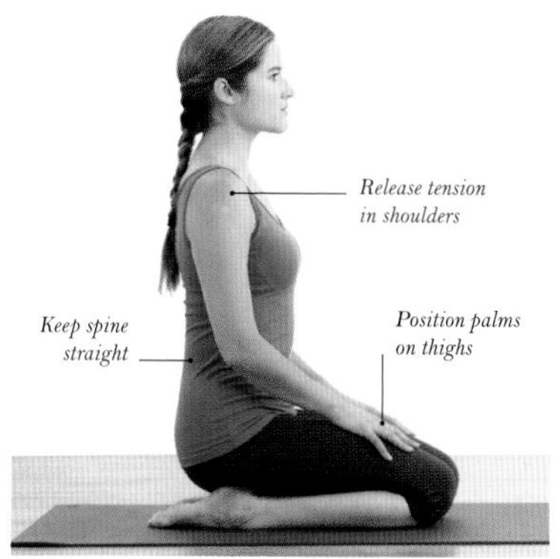

49 PLANK

The Plank pose is an all-around strengthening posture. But it is also ideal for releasing stress in the neck, as well as for lengthening the spine.

1 Sit with your legs folded under yourself and with your toes pointing away. Put your hands on your thighs, fingers pointing forward. Straighten your neck and back, keeping your chin parallel to the floor. Allow your breath to flow in and out easily.

2 Position yourself on all fours, keeping your knees hip-width apart and directly under your hips. Your arms should be parallel to your thighs, and your back flat. Pull in your abdomen.

Pull abdomen in
toward spine
Hold knees
hip-width apart
Keep soles of
feet upward
Hold arms
shoulder-width
apart

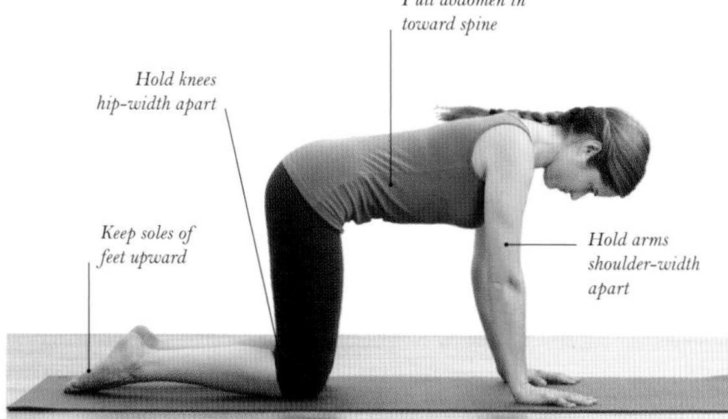

3 As you breathe in, extend your legs, locking your knees and elbows and keeping your body straight. Grip the mat with your toes, and push your heels back. Hold for as long as you are able, then release.

Keep knees
locked
Keep arms
straight
Spread fingers
and root down
through fingertips

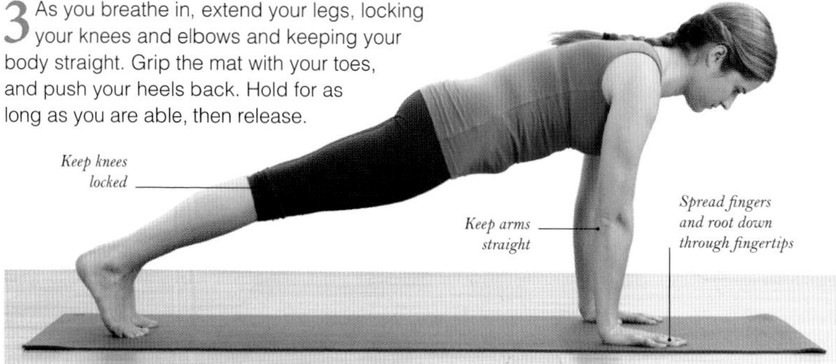

50 LEG RAISE

Elevating the leg provides a strong stretch to the hamstring and calf muscles. This pose develops the flexibility and strength needed for forward-bending poses. Begin by raising each leg three times, synchronizing each movement with your breath.

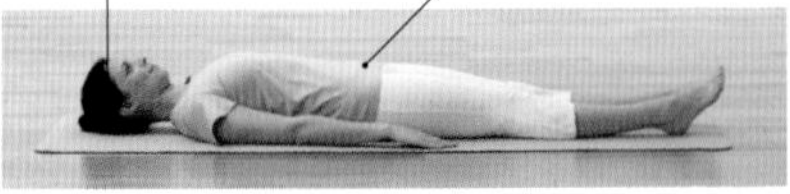

Keep head centered

Breathe from abdomen

1 Lie flat on your back with your feet together and your arms on the floor at your sides, palms down. Flex your feet slightly.

2 Inhale as you raise your left leg, then exhale as you lower it. Repeat this action for the right leg. Complete five sets of raises.

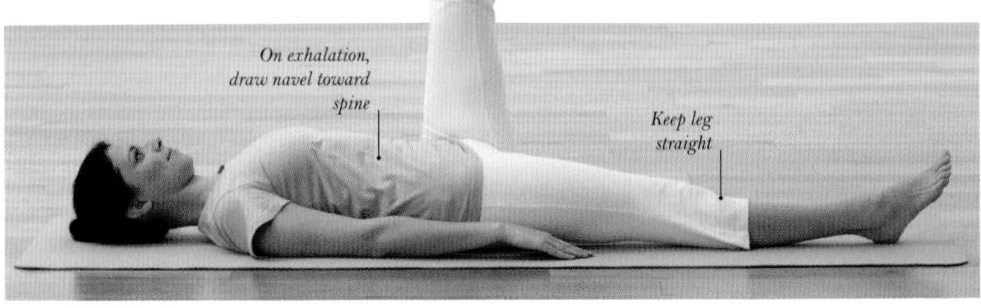

51 LEG RAISE 2

In this alternative version of the Leg Raise, you draw the head toward the knee to compress the abdomen. Consequently, this particular exercise strengthens the neck, abdominal, and lumbar muscles. It also helps tone the legs.

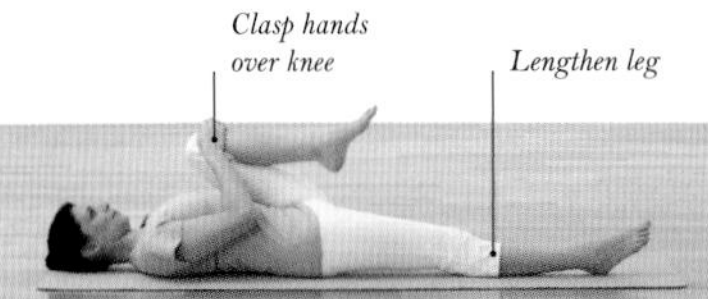

1 Lie flat on your back. As you exhale, bend your left leg, bringing the knee into your chest. Take the knee in both hands to help press your left thigh to the abdomen.

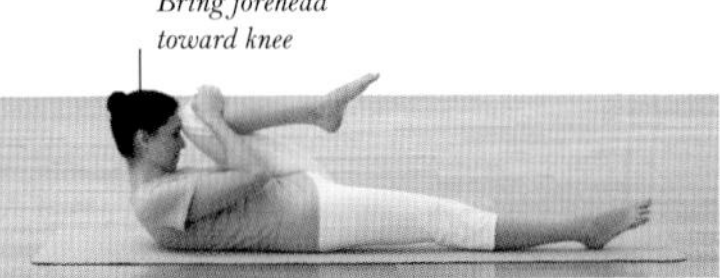

2 As you inhale, lift your head toward the knee. Then exhale, slowly lowering head, arms, and leg. Repeat with the right leg. Complete the whole exercise five times.

52

TRIANGLE

This posture is excellent for building strength in the back and core. It also helps improve the flexibility of the hip joints and opens up the chest.

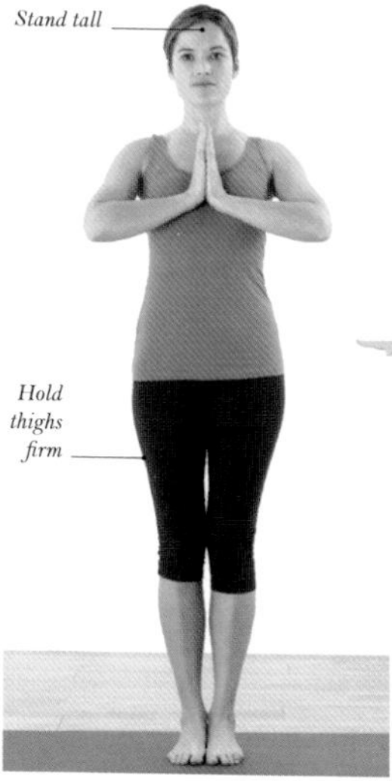

Stand tall

Hold thighs firm

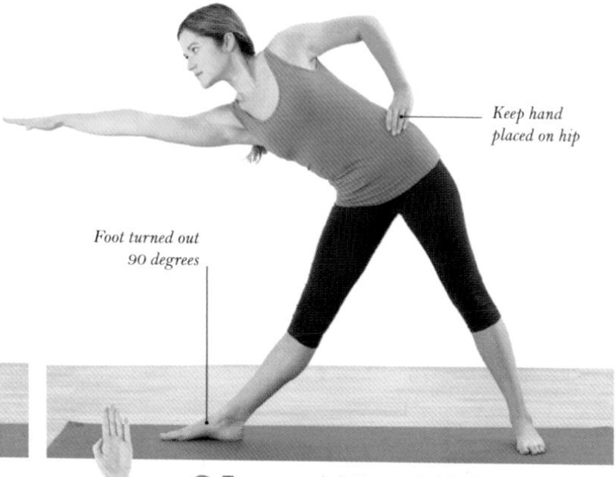

Keep hand placed on hip

Foot turned out 90 degrees

1 Stand with feet together and hands in prayer pose, and focus on your breathing. Jump or walk your feet 3 ft (1 m) apart, with toes forward and knees locked.

2 Turn your right leg out. Inhale, and raise your arms to shoulder level with your palms facing downward, then place your left hand on your hip. As you exhale, pivot from the hip to the right. Breathe into the stretch.

3 Exhale to bring your right arm down to rest on or behind your right leg, depending on comfort, and extend your left arm straight up. Hold the pose for several breaths. Reverse the movement to release, then repeat on the left side.

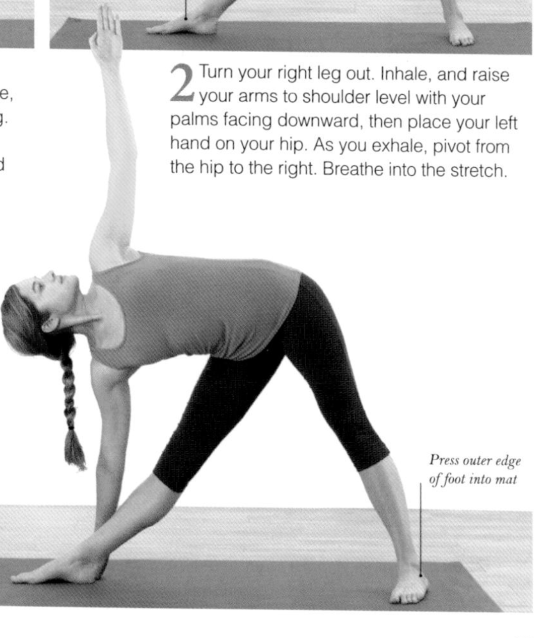

Press outer edge of foot into mat

53 WARRIOR

The Warrior asana helps strengthen the mind as well as the body. Keep the lower part of the body firmly grounded while allowing the upper body the freedom to move with control and purpose.

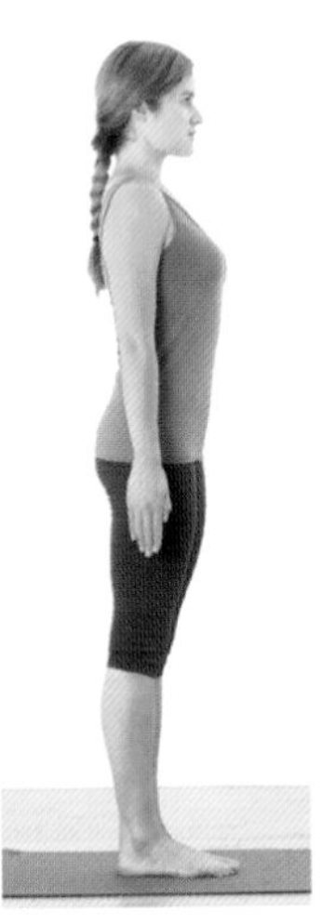

1 Start in step 1 of the Mountain Pose (see p.30). Lengthen your spine, and breathe in a gentle rhythm.

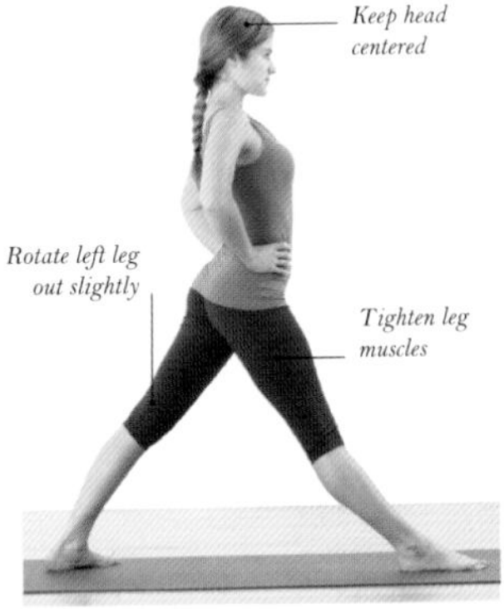

Keep head centered

Rotate left leg out slightly

Tighten leg muscles

2 Exhaling, step forward with your right foot as far as is comfortable. Put your hands on your hips, which should face forward, and lock your knees. Angle your left foot out to about 60 degrees.

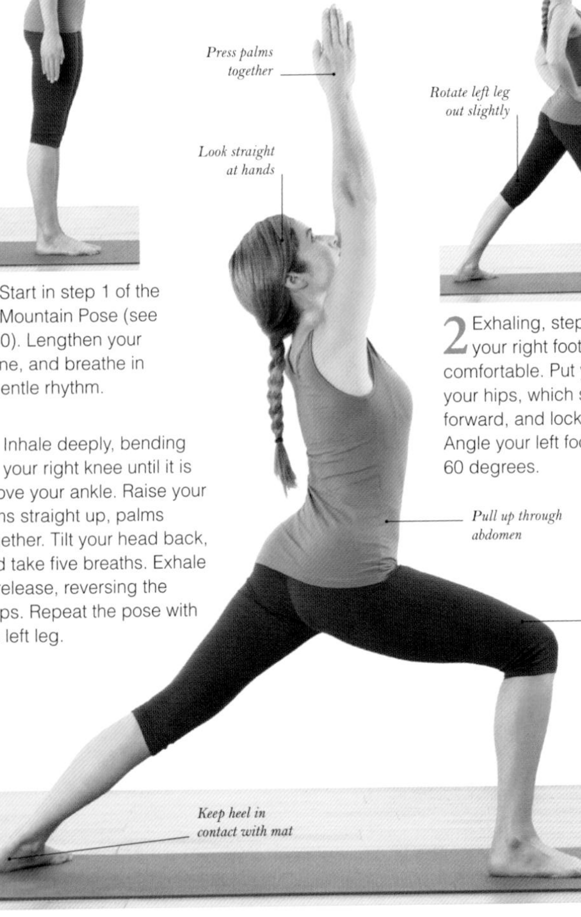

Press palms together

Look straight at hands

Pull up through abdomen

Knee should be above ankle

Keep heel in contact with mat

3 Inhale deeply, bending your right knee until it is above your ankle. Raise your arms straight up, palms together. Tilt your head back, and take five breaths. Exhale to release, reversing the steps. Repeat the pose with the left leg.

54 WARRIOR LUNGE

This posture really works the quadriceps, which are the muscles at the front of your thighs, as well as gently stretching your lower back.

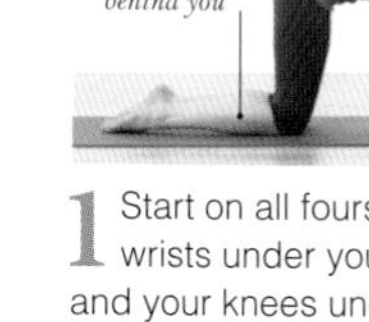

1 Start on all fours, with your wrists under your shoulders and your knees under your hips. Draw your navel toward the spine to flatten the back.

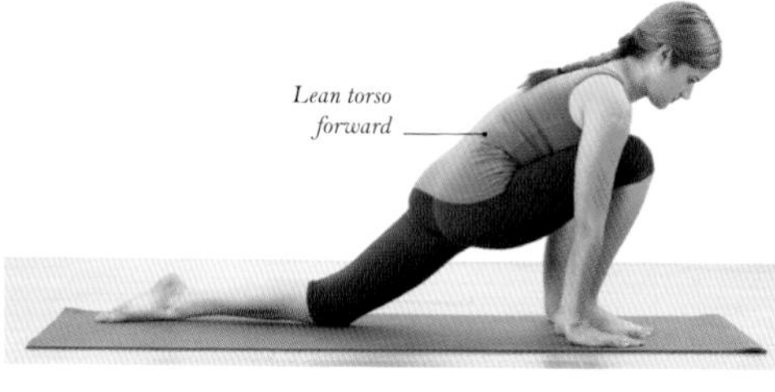

2 Exhaling, bring your right foot next to your right thumb. At the same time, lean forward at a 45-degree angle, so the right side of your abdomen is next to the right thigh.

3 Raise your torso slightly by lifting your hands, keeping the fingers pressed into the mat. Lift your left knee and turn your toes under to take the weight.

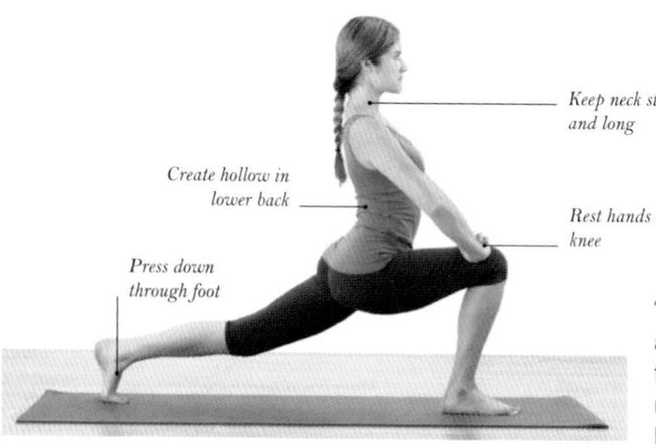

4 Lift your hands onto your right knee. Look forward and straighten your torso. Hold for five breaths. On exhalation, release and return to all fours. Repeat on the other side.

55 WARRIOR 2

This variant of the Warrior pose helps tone the abdomen, as well as strengthening the limbs and opening the chest and shoulders. Start off in step 2 of Mountain Pose (see p.30). Focus on your breathing, and center yourself, then jump or walk your feet out so they are about 3 ft (1 m) apart.

Right leg faces forward
Left leg turned out 90 degrees

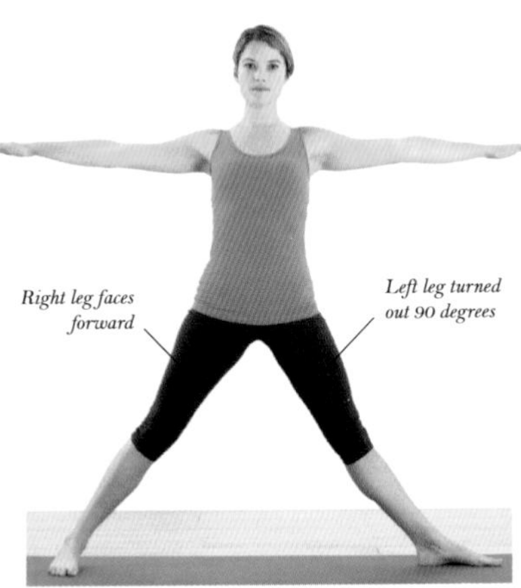

1 Breathe in and as you do so, raise your arms up, palms down, level with your shoulders. Turn your left foot until it is pointing in the same direction as your left hand. Keep the right foot facing forward.

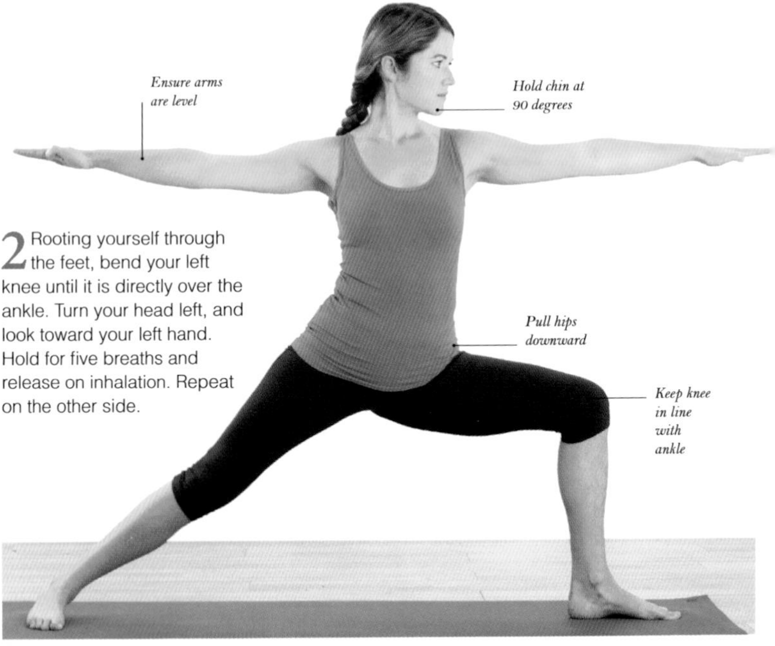

Ensure arms are level

Hold chin at 90 degrees

2 Rooting yourself through the feet, bend your left knee until it is directly over the ankle. Turn your head left, and look toward your left hand. Hold for five breaths and release on inhalation. Repeat on the other side.

Pull hips downward

Keep knee in line with ankle

56 DOWNWARD-FACING DOG

This is one of the best-known of all yoga postures, and for good reason. As well as being perfect for energizing the entire body, it also helps calm the mind and gives a strong stretch in the shoulders, hamstrings, and calves. Begin on all fours with hands shoulder-width apart and knees hip-width apart.

Draw navel toward spine on exhalation

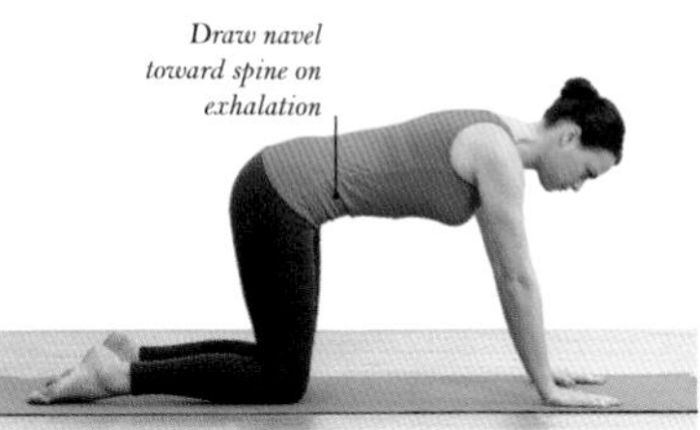

1 Move your hands slightly ahead of your shoulders, spreading your fingers so that your middle fingers are pointing forward.

Draw back your hips
Keep your back flat
Keep arms straight

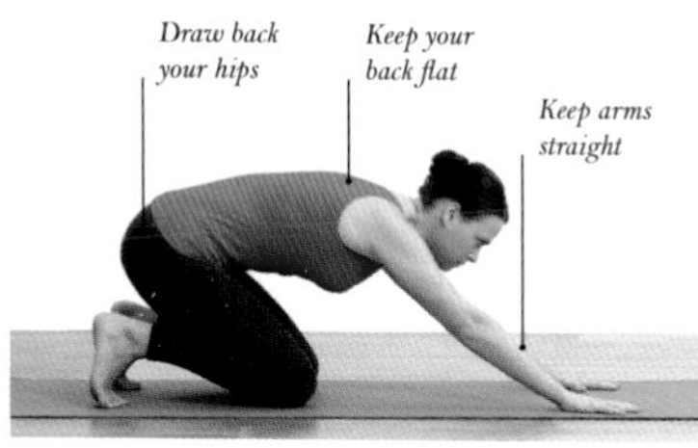

2 Turn your toes under your feet, keeping the soles vertical to the floor, and draw your hips back toward your feet.

Bring tailbone upward
Spread toes and root down
Keep neck relaxed

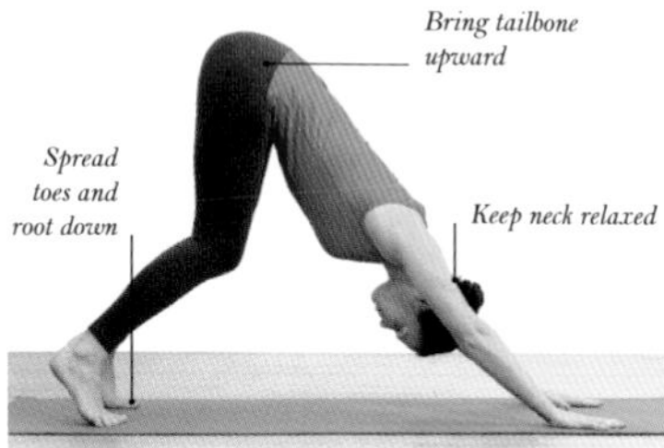

3 As you exhale, lift your knees, drawing your tailbone up. Keep the knees slightly bent and your heels off the floor.

4 Straighten your arms and legs as much as you are able, and push back into your heels. Relax your neck, and breathe evenly. Every time you exhale, lengthen your spine.

Extend your back
Be aware of movement of abdomen
Keep head in line with body
Stretch backs of legs
Spread fingers to reduce pressure on wrists
Flatten feet to floor

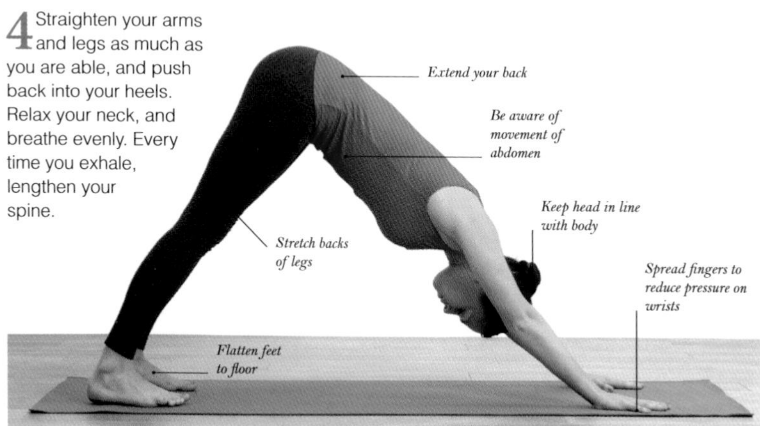

57 EXTENDED SIDE STRETCH

Use this posture to help tone and strengthen your legs, improve lung capacity, and stimulate the organs in the abdomen.

Extend arms fully
Turn left foot in slightly

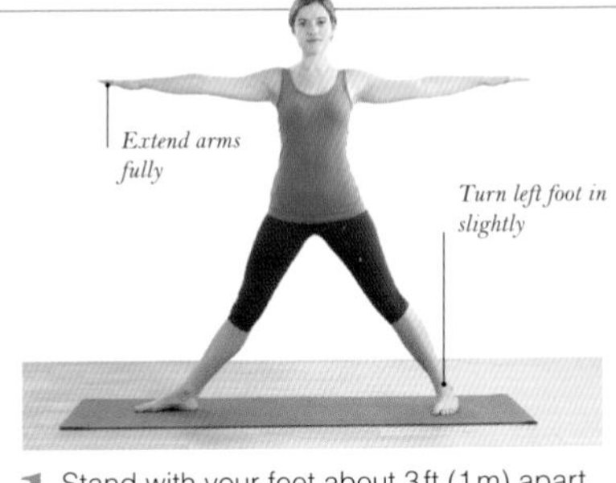

1 Stand with your feet about 3 ft (1 m) apart. As you inhale, raise your arms parallel to the floor, palms down. Turn your left foot in slightly and your right foot out to 90 degrees.

Turn head right to 90 degrees

Keep knee above ankle

2 Exhale, bending your right knee until it is above your right ankle. Keeping your arms parallel to the floor, stretch them out wide, locked at the elbows. Try also to bring the right thigh parallel to the floor.

Keep hips open

3 Exhale to lean your upper body forward, with the right forearm on your thigh. Bring your left hand into the small of your back.

Arm is in line with leg
Exhale to extend further
Keep knee at 90 degrees
Root down through right foot

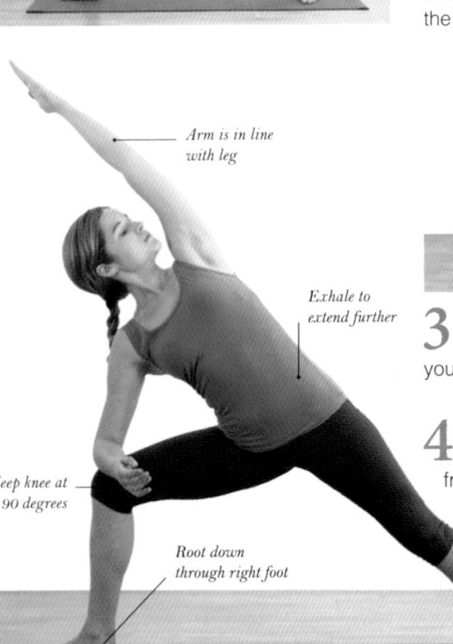

4 Extend your left arm up and over the back of your left ear, palm down. Stretch from the left heel up to your left fingertips. Look up at your left arm. Inhale and straighten the front leg to release. Repeat on the other side.

58 HALF SPINAL TWIST

This pose involves a lateral twist along the complete length of the spine. It helps increase your spinal flexibility and therefore benefits overall posture. It is also useful for releasing tension throughout the body. Complete the exercise on both sides.

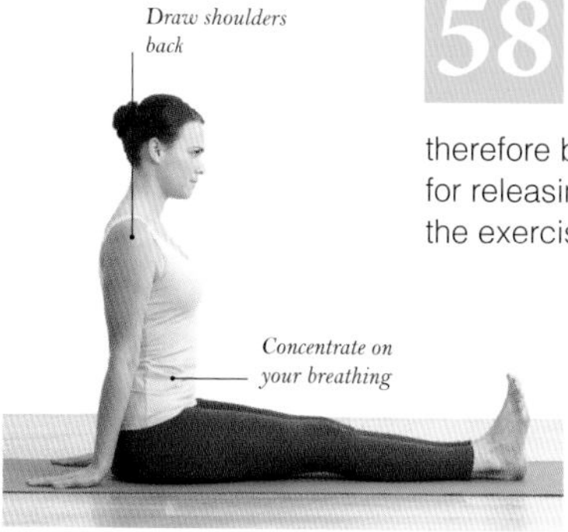

Draw shoulders back

Concentrate on your breathing

1 Sit with your back straight and your legs extended. Keeping your arms straight, place your palms on the mat behind you, with fingers pointing away from your body. Breathe from the abdomen.

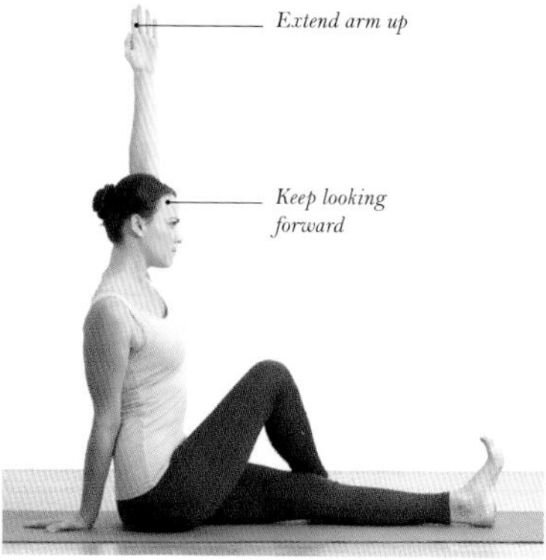

Extend arm up

Keep looking forward

2 Bring your right foot to the mat over your left leg, next to your left calf. As you inhale, lift your left arm straight up, palm open and fingers extended.

Turn head 90 degrees right

3 Exhale, bringing the left elbow to the outside of the right knee, palm to the right. Lift upward from the waist, then twist until you are looking over your right shoulder. Breathe slowly from the abdomen.

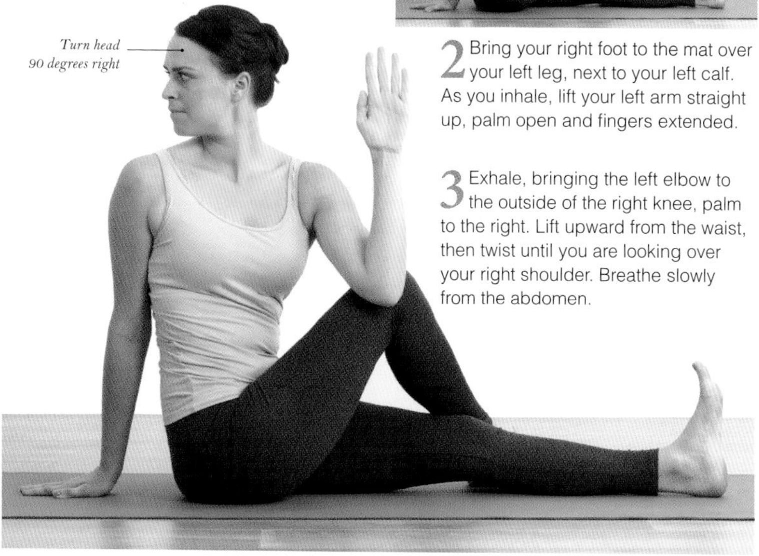

59 HORSE

This pose helps strengthen the core and stretch the leg muscles. It also lengthens the spine and opens the hips, making it particularly good for combating the effects of prolonged sitting.

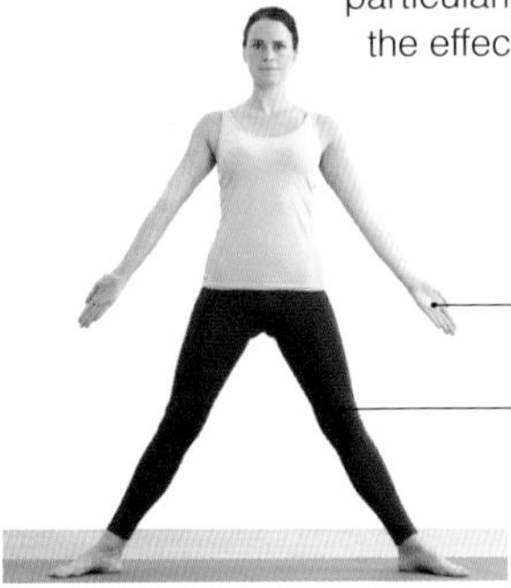

Arms raised to 45 degrees

Keep feet about 3ft (1 m) apart

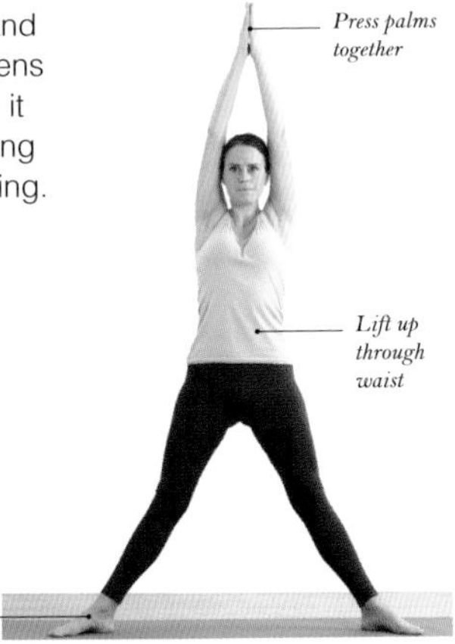

1 Start with your feet about 3ft (1m) apart and turned outward to 45 degrees. Inhale and raise the arms 45 degrees, palms forward.

Press palms together

Lift up through waist

Feet pressed into mat

2 Firm your leg muscles, and inhale slowly, sweeping the arms up until the palms are together above the head, arms fully extended.

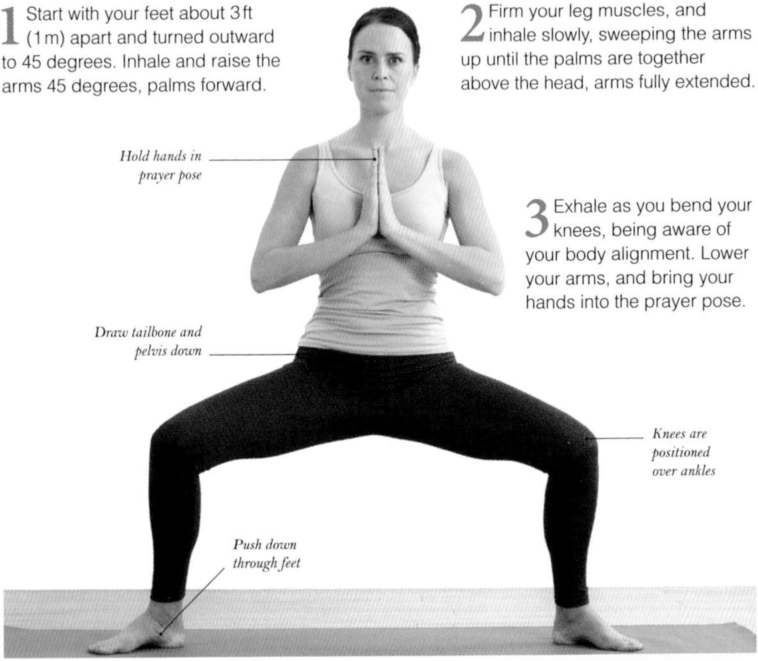

Hold hands in prayer pose

Draw tailbone and pelvis down

Knees are positioned over ankles

Push down through feet

3 Exhale as you bend your knees, being aware of your body alignment. Lower your arms, and bring your hands into the prayer pose.

60 COBRA

This is a face-down pose that requires that you lift the upper body, curling up and back like a cobra. By holding the posture, you tone and strengthen the muscles of the back and abdomen. It also increases the flexibility of your spine and helps relieve tension.

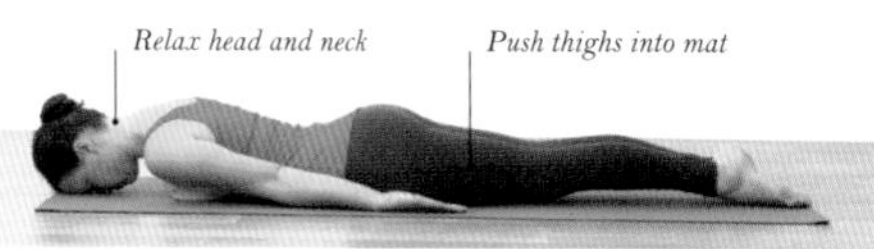

1 Lie face down, with your forehead resting on the mat and your arms by your sides, palms up. Stretch your legs, and point your toes away from your body.

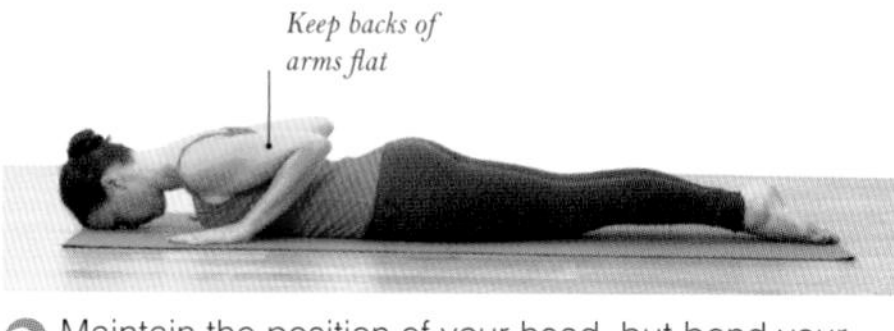

2 Maintain the position of your head, but bend your arms in order to bring the palms of your hands flat on the floor, on each side of your chest.

3 Take a deep breath in, and raise your head and chest, arching the spine and pressing your shoulder blades together. Hold for five to ten breaths, then return to the starting position.

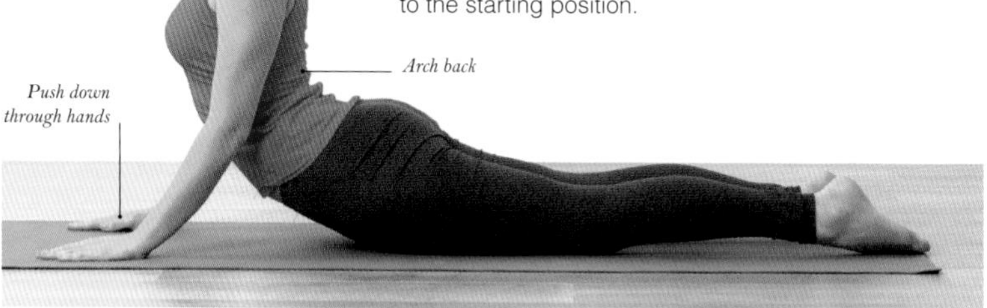

61 PURPOSE OF THE SUN SALUTATION

The Sun Salutation (see overleaf) is a graceful, fluid 12-step routine that brings together several poses to loosen up body and mind in preparation for your yoga session. The positions employed are tied into your breathing pattern, helping instill a feeling of balance and harmony. Furthermore, the order in which the postures are put together leads to a variety of beneficial spinal movements. Once you know the routine, try to complete the Sun Salutation at least six times before each yoga session.

SUN SALUTATION

Traditionally performed to greet the rising sun, this sequence of postures helps warm the muscles, flex the spine, and synchronize the breathing with the movement of the body.

Keep arms apart as they rise
Align head, neck, and back
Ensure shoulders are relaxed
Bend forward from hips
Start with hands at your sides
Bend knees slightly if necessary

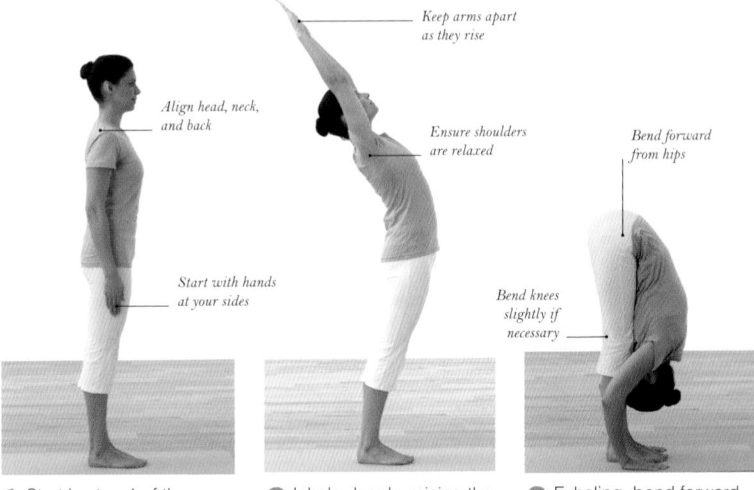

1 Start in step 1 of the Mountain Pose (see p.30). As you breathe out, bring your hands up into the prayer position.

2 Inhale deeply, raising the arms, palms forward, and bend back from the waist, pushing out your hips and keeping the legs straight.

3 Exhaling, bend forward from the hips, and place the palms beside your feet. They stay in this position for the rest of the sequence.

4 As you breathe in, stretch your left leg backward as far as you can, and rest your left knee on the floor. Bring your shoulder blades together, and press down through your fingertips. Arch your back by tilting your face upward.

Stretch head upward
Extend leg back
Stretch your foot

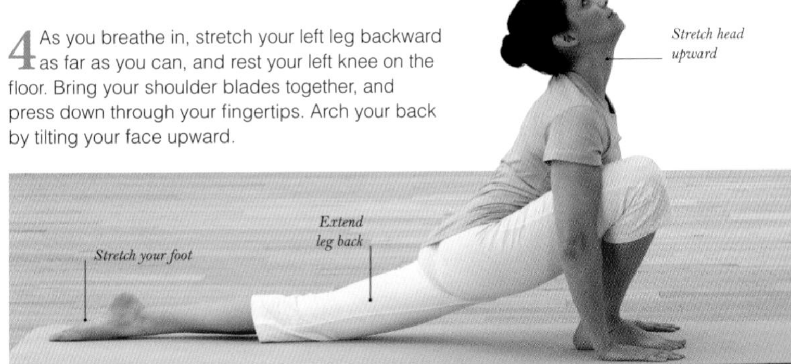

Press toes
into mat
Do not raise or
drop hips
Keep elbows
straight

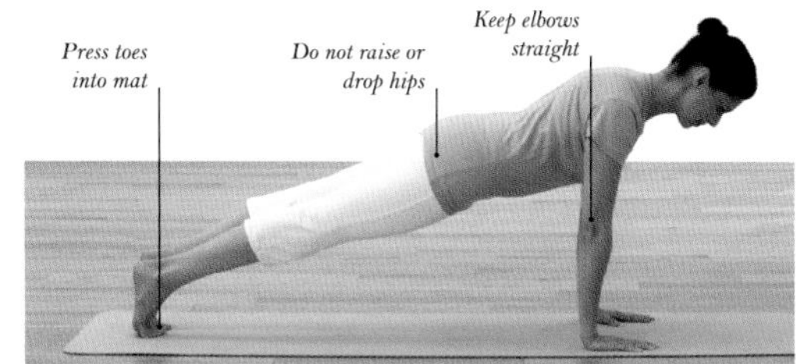

5 Hold your breath as you bring your right foot back and move onto your toes so that your entire body is in a straight, inclined line.

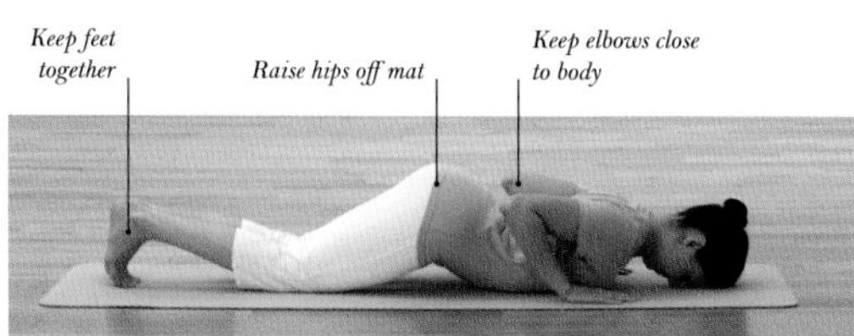

6 Exhale, lowering your knees to the floor and your chest straight down between your hands, touching your forehead to the mat. Keep your hips raised up.

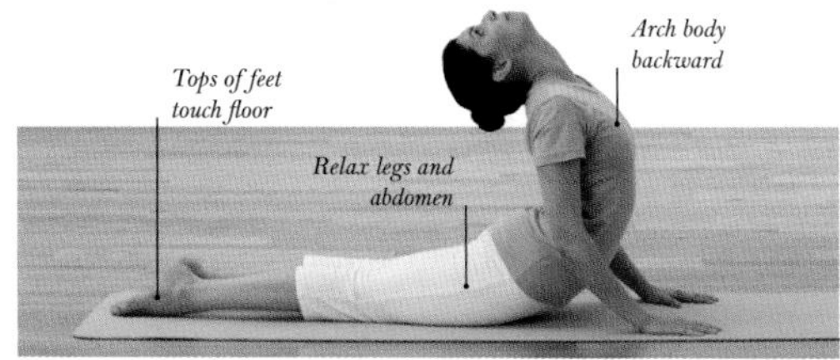

7 Inhale, lowering your hips and extending your feet backward. Arch your spine to look upward, pushing your chest forward. Keep your abdomen and legs relaxed.

Lengthen tailbone
away from pelvis
Keep back as
straight as
possible
Lengthen
through arms

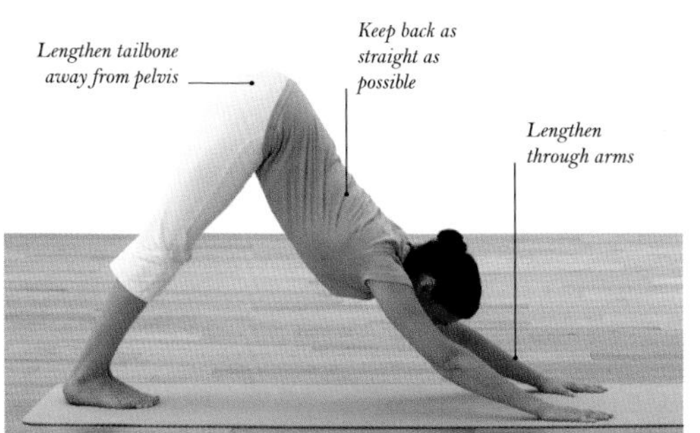

8 Exhale and turn your toes under, raising your hips to make an inverted V-shape. Push your hips back as far as possible. Keep your back straight and heels pressed down.

ENDING THE SUN SALUTATION
The last four steps of the Sun Salutation are essentially repeats of earlier poses. From step 8, move into the position in step 4 but on the other side of the body—by bringing your left leg forward instead of back. From this lunge posture, you then work backward through steps 3, 2, and 1, although excluding the prayer pose.

POSES FOR TONE & STRETCH

HOW YOGA IMPROVES BODY TONE

In yoga, muscles are worked dynamically—that is, stretched and strengthened at the same time, which is perfect for muscle tone. Regular practice will lead to greater definition as the muscles become lean and toned. When your strength and flexibility have built up, you can make your practice even more intense by holding poses for longer or by moving more swiftly between asanas. Muscle tone can also be increased through varying the choice of postures in your yoga sessions.

64 STANDING FORWARD BEND

The chief benefit of this asana is the intense stretch that it gives you—from the middle of your back, all the way down your legs to your heels. Once you are in the final position, hold it for several breaths, lengthening the lower back and leg muscles with each.

Hold arms at your sides

Tune in to your breathing

Stand with feet hip-width apart

1 Stand in step 1 of Mountain pose (see p30). Center yourself, and focus on your breath as you root down.

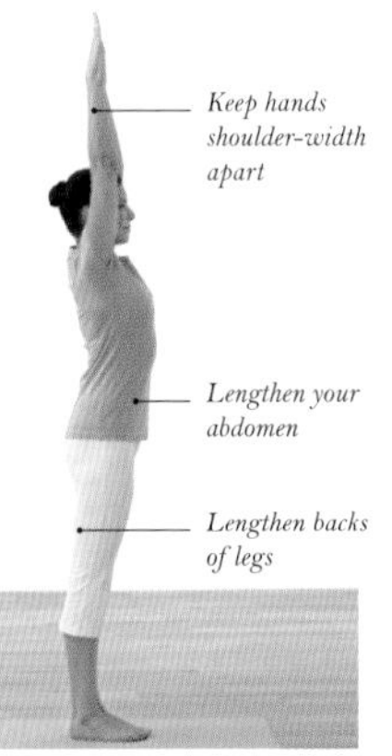

2 Inhale deeply, lock your arms at the elbow and slowly sweep them up. Tilt your head to look up at your hands.

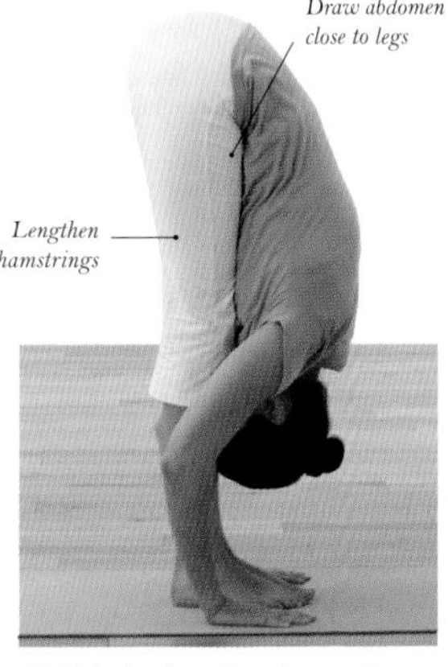

3 Exhale, bending forward from the hips, bringing your fingertips to the floor. Lengthen the backs of the legs and place your palms next to your feet.

LEGS UP THE WALL POSE

In this posture, the upper body is supported completely by the floor, while the wall partially supports your legs, helping their upward extension. This is an ideal asana as preparation for more advanced inverted poses.

Position shoulder against wall
Place hands on thighs

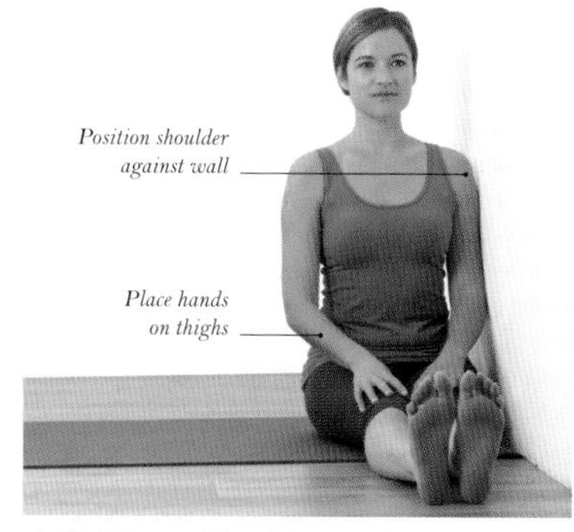

1 Sit fully upright with your left hip and shoulder pressed against the wall. Place your palms on top of your thighs.

Use hands to help stabilize yourself

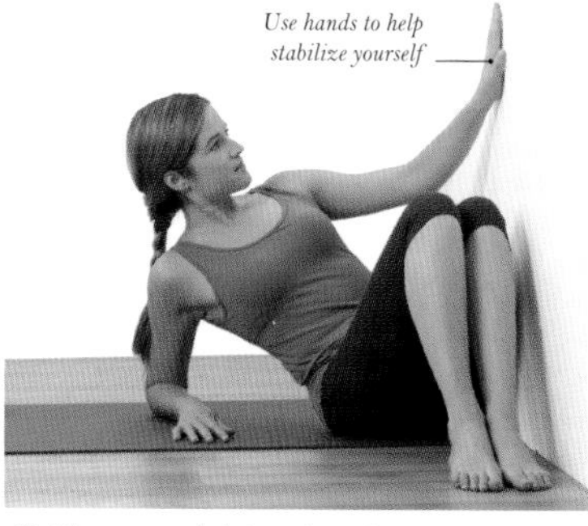

2 Place your left hand against the wall, then lean back, lowering yourself down onto your right elbow, and draw up your knees.

3 Extend your legs up the wall and keep your back flat on the floor, with your hands on your stomach. Keep your legs and heels pressed against the wall, and hold the pose for several breaths.

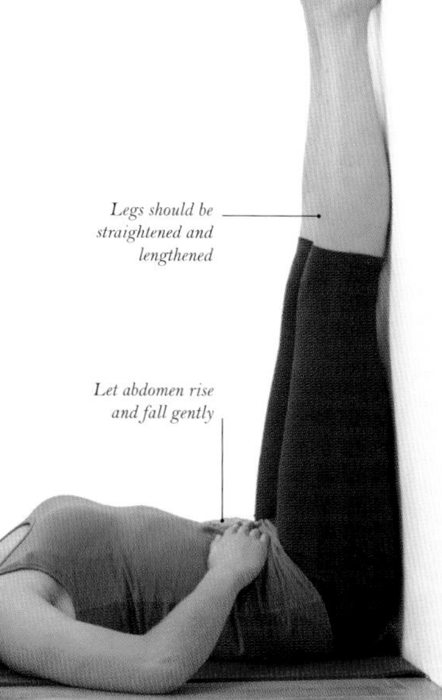

66 BRIDGE POSE

This backward-bend asana promotes relaxation and can help with the reduction of stress. It stretches the spine and the thoracic and lumbar regions, but it is also a good posture to carry out when your feet are feeling tired.

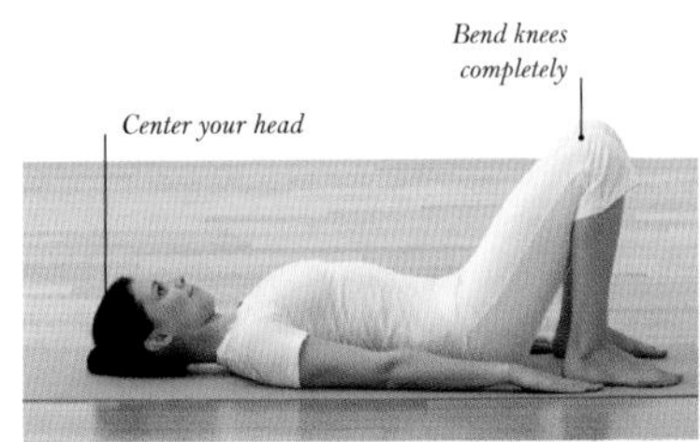

1 Position yourself on your back, with your knees bent and your feet flat on the floor, close to your behind. Extend your arms, palms down, alongside your body.

Feet are hip-width apart
Push hips up to arch back

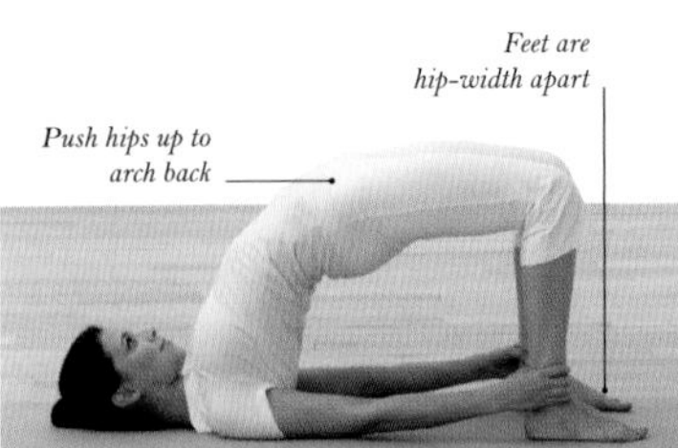

2 Edge the hands to the feet and hold the heels or ankles. Keep your feet firm. Inhale, pushing your hips up and arching the spine to lift the lower back clear of the floor.

Use hands to support back
Keeps legs slightly apart
Keep head centered

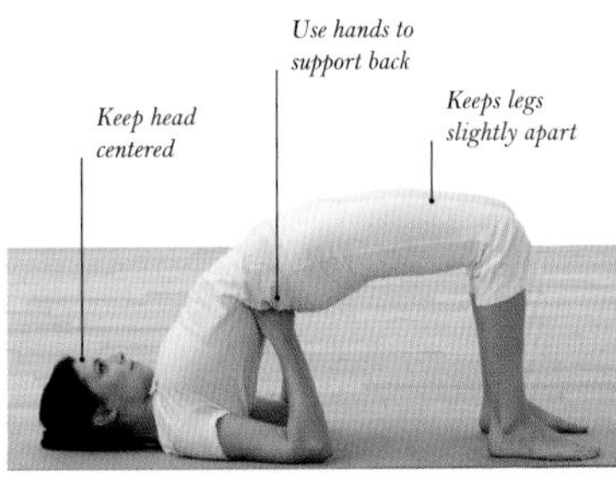

3 Release your feet. Keeping your upper arms planted, place your hands as high up your back as you can. Take a few deep breaths before reversing the steps to release.

BRIDGE VARIATIONS

If you would like more of a challenge, these variations on the Bridge work different muscle groups.

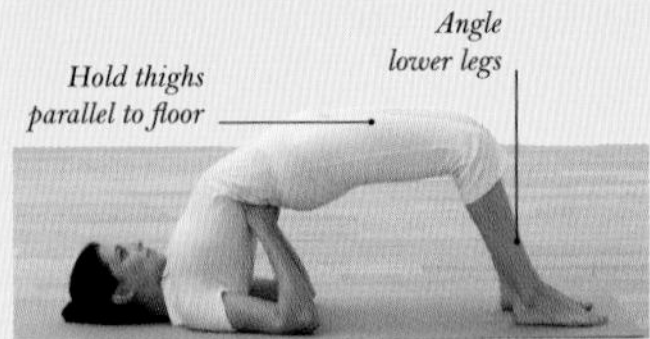

Hamstring stretch variation
Once in the Bridge posture, take several deep breaths. Edge your feet away from you to create a 45-degree angle to the floor with your lower legs.

Extend foot, pointing toes up
Keep raised leg perpendicular to floor
Thigh parallel to floor

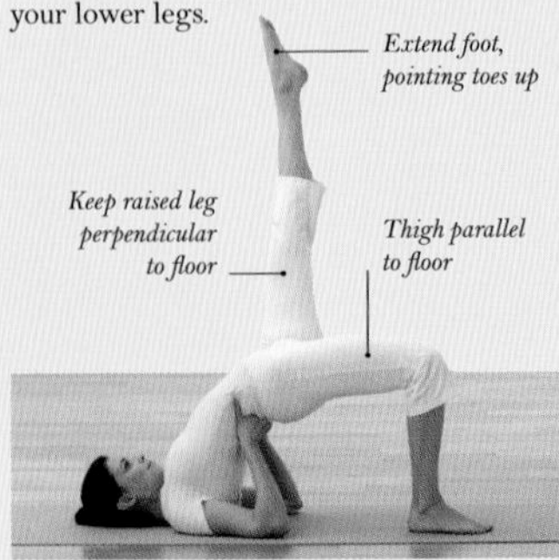

Leg lift variation
From the Bridge pose, raise your left leg 90 degrees to the floor and point your foot. Take five breaths, then release on exhalation. Repeat on the right.

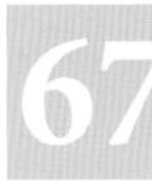

COBBLER

This posture is good for stress relief because it helps release tension in the hips, legs, and lower back. Additionally, it opens up the hips and improves circulation.

Center your head
Pull back shoulders

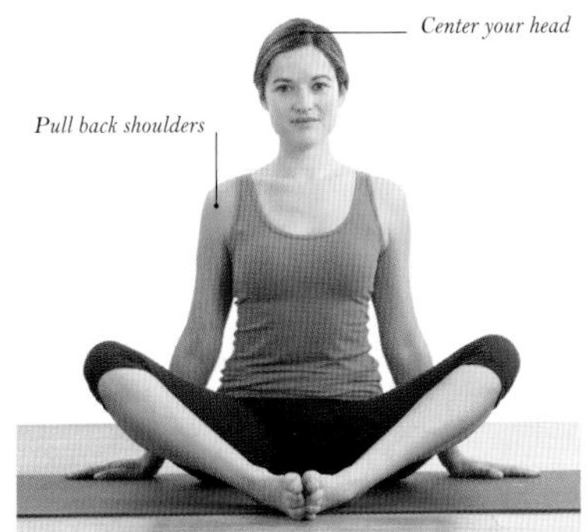

1 Sit with your legs straight out in front of you and hands by your sides. Bend your knees and draw your feet together, positioning them sole to sole. Keep your back straight.

Allow face to relax
Bring arms to front

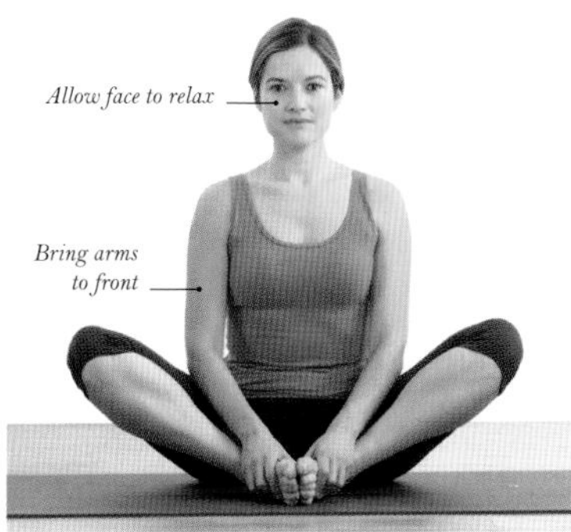

2 Keeping your feet pressed together, bring your hands around and take a firm hold of them. Your head should remain centered and your spine lengthened.

Focus on your breathing
Push knees down gently

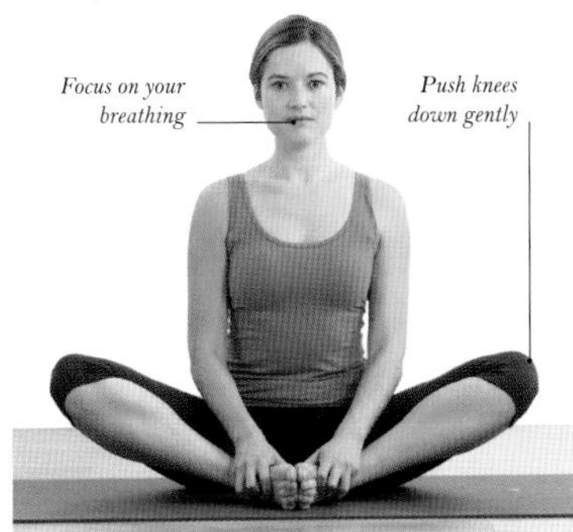

3 On an outward breath, gently extend your knees, bringing them out and down toward the mat, letting the hips open. Continue to elongate the spine.

Rest hands on knees

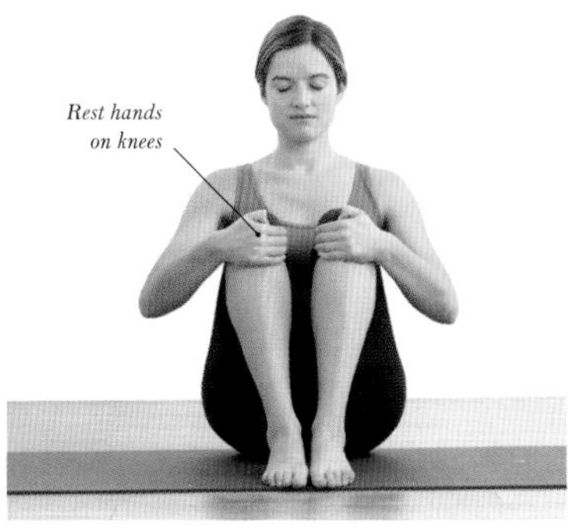

4 To end, slowly move the knees up toward your chest, then run your hands up from feet to knees. Rock from side to side, feeling the stretch in your hips.

68 SITTING FORWARD STRETCH

When you need to calm your mind, this is a great go-to asana. It also stretches the hamstrings and the spine, as well as massaging the abdominal organs.

Position foot using both hands

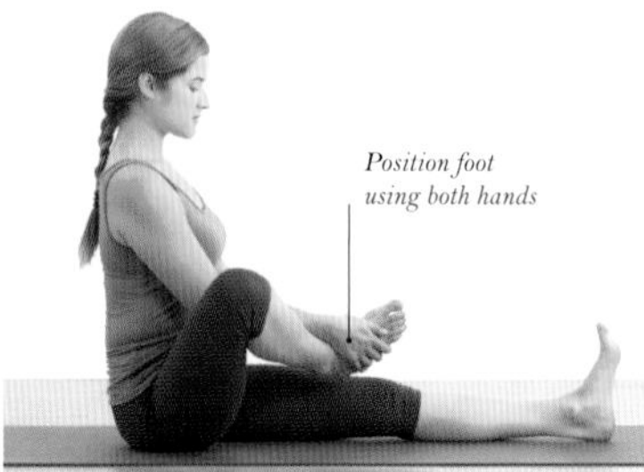

1 Sit with legs extended in front of you. As you inhale, bend your right leg. Take hold of the foot, and bring the heel toward you.

Raise arms to vertical position
Inhale as you lift arms

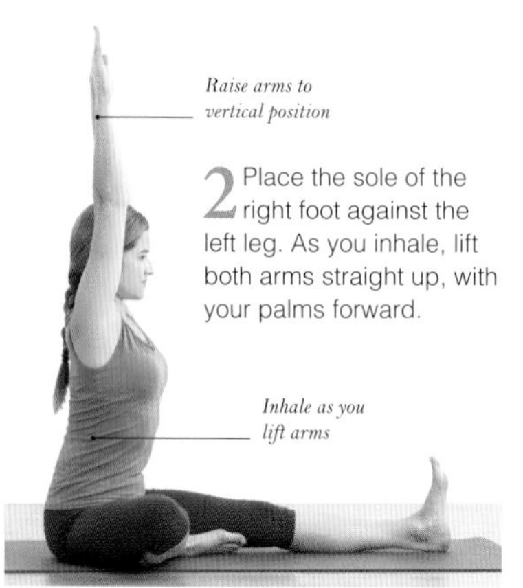

2 Place the sole of the right foot against the left leg. As you inhale, lift both arms straight up, with your palms forward.

Keep head aligned with back
Bring arms forward

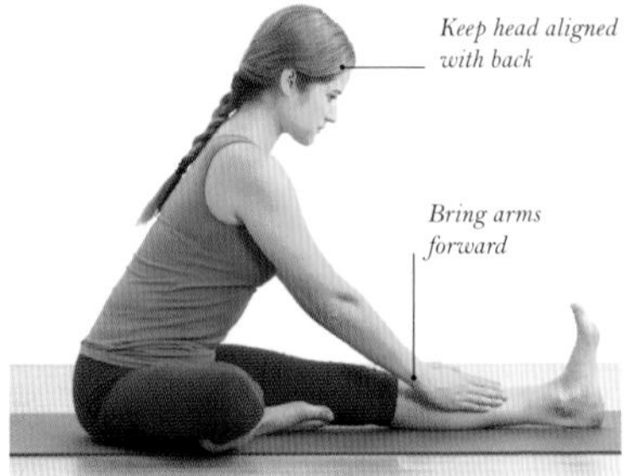

3 On the outward breath, bring your arms to rest on your left shin, bending from the waist. Inhale, stretching through the spine.

4 Exhale, bringing your torso toward your extended leg. Breathe in slowly as you sit back up. Repeat on the other side.

Relax your hips
Hold foot if possible

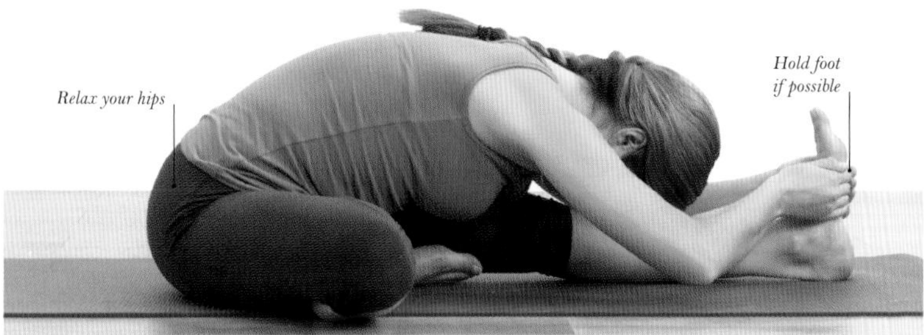

69 EXTENDED SITTING STRETCH

By extending the spine, arms, and legs all at the same time, this posture helps prepare you for other sitting stretch poses that you might include in your session.

Look straight ahead
Toes flexed toward torso

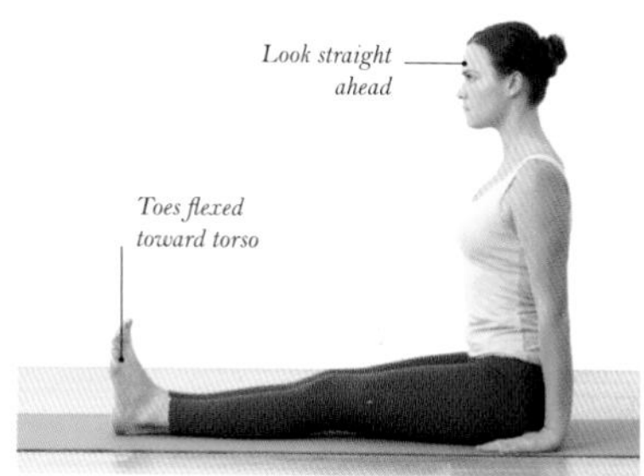

1 Sit with your legs extended in front of you, elbows locked, and palms pressed down. Breathe in deeply to lift and expand the chest.

Raise arms with palms forward initially
Fully extend legs

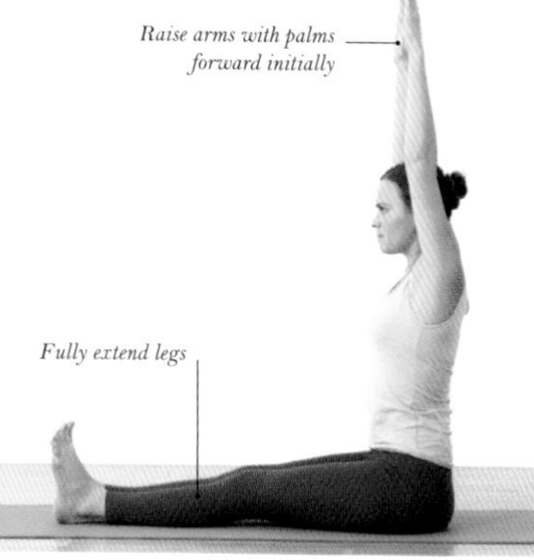

2 With your back upright, inhale and lift your arms. Press the palms together, interlock the fingers, and turn the palms up. Stretch up, and hold for five breaths. Release and lower.

3 Repeat step 2, this time interlocking your fingers the less natural way, so the little finger that was on top is now underneath.

Fingers are interlocked
Keep head centered
Lengthen legs by pushing heels away from you

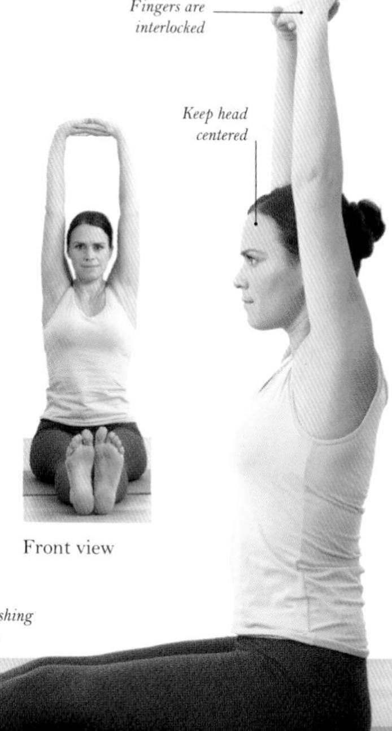

Front view

70 CAT POSE

As well as strengthening the lower-back muscles, the Cat gives the spine and abdominal organs a gentle massage. By stretching the back, torso, and neck, it is also a good stress-relieving asana.

Keep your back straight
Relaxed neck
Thighs at 90° to floor

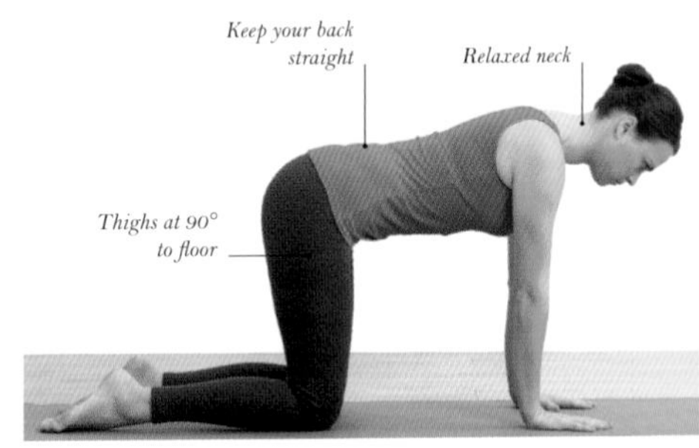

1 Start on all fours, with wrists under the shoulders and knees under the hips. Point the toes away from the body. Flatten your back by drawing the navel up to the spine.

Spine curves down on inhalation

Stretch neck to look forward

2 As you breathe in, gently curve the spine down by pulling the tailbone up and pushing the chest out. Raise your chin and look up.

3 Exhale, lowering the tailbone and raising the abdomen, creating an upward arch in the spine. Drop your head between your arms without exerting any downward force on it.

Back is arched
Draw down crown of head
Abdomen is raised
Stabilize yourself through palms

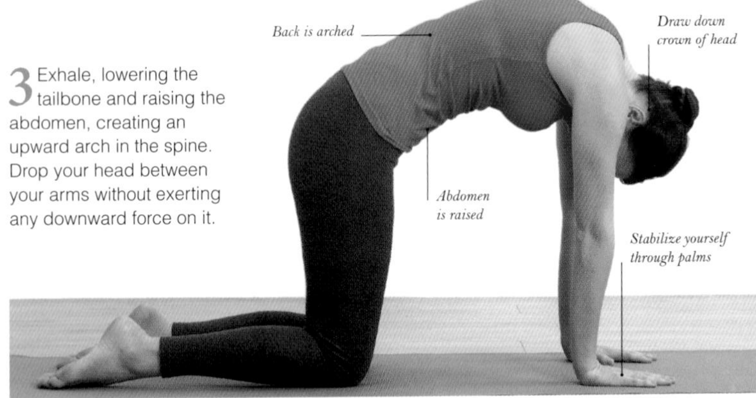

71 LUNGE TWIST

Practice this asana to help tone and strengthen the muscles in the upper legs. It is also a recommended posture for improving the flexibility of the spine. Come out of step 4 after a few breaths by reversing the process, then repeat on the other side.

Back is naturally curved
Spread fingers to help with stability

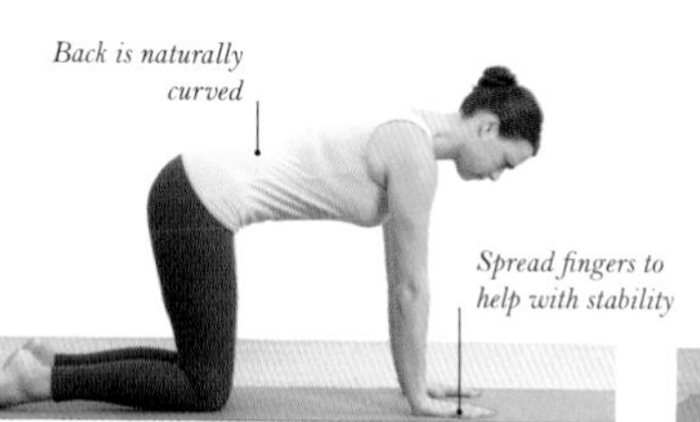

1 Begin on your hands and knees, with your arms shoulder-width apart and your legs hip-width apart. Look down at your fingers.

Head is centered
Relax your shoulders
Arm extended with palm open
Rotate torso
Knee brought back over ankle

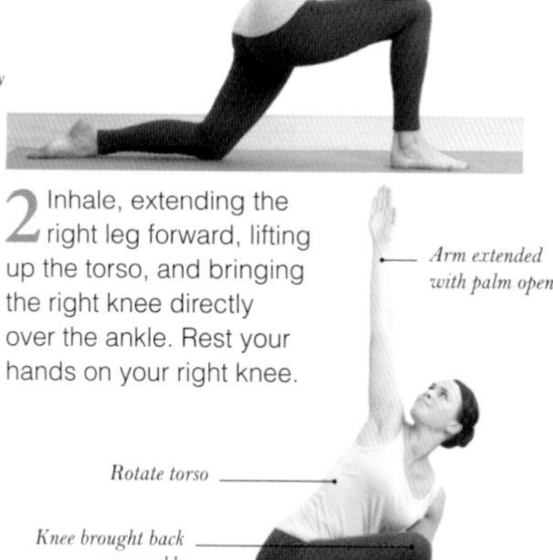

2 Inhale, extending the right leg forward, lifting up the torso, and bringing the right knee directly over the ankle. Rest your hands on your right knee.

Lengthen through spine
Press top of foot into mat

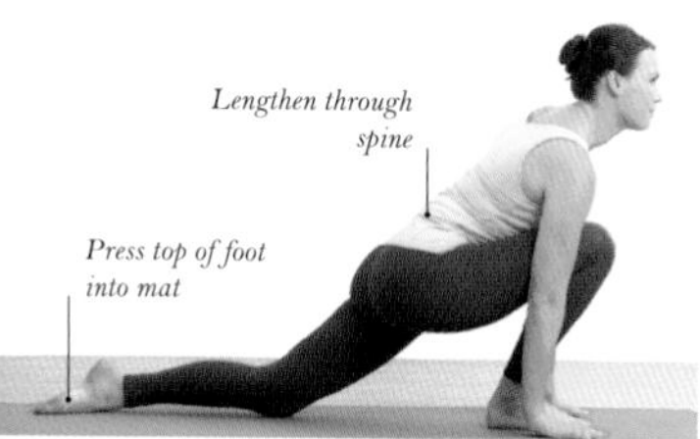

3 Keeping your feet static, inhale as you lean forward, increasing the right-knee bend. Place a hand on each side of the right foot.

4 On an out breath, push the left hand into the mat, then lift your right arm up to point at the ceiling. Look at the raised hand.

LUNGE TWIST VARIATION

In this variation on (and addition to) step 4, you bring your left elbow over and across the right knee and lower the right arm to come into the prayer pose. Turn your head to look up, until your chin is over the right shoulder. On exhalation, try to open the chest and rotate the torso.

Hands in prayer pose
Head turned 90° from center

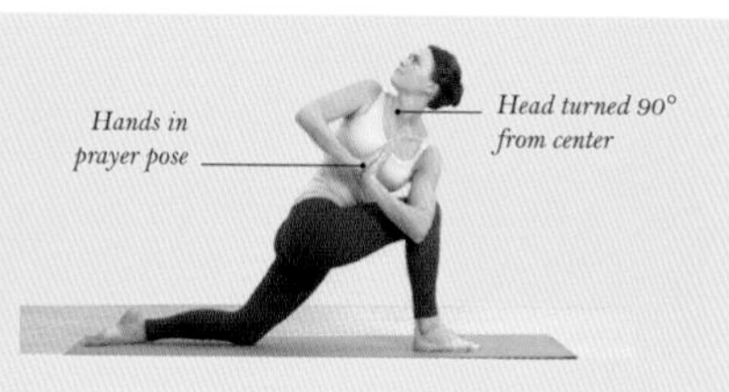

72 SEATED FORWARD BEND

Although it looks like an easy posture, when it is performed correctly, the Seated Forward Bend can work wonders on your hamstring muscles and spine.

1 Sit with your back and arms straight, palms flat on the mat and your legs stretched out in front of you. Point your feet up, and flex the toes slightly.

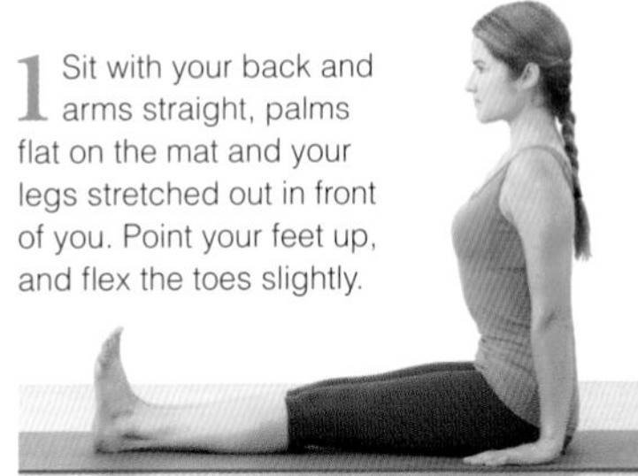

SIMPLIFIED FORM

People who are not flexible enough to reach their ankles can still practice this exercise. Place a strap around the balls of both feet and bring your hands as close to your feet as you are able when bending forward with a straight back.

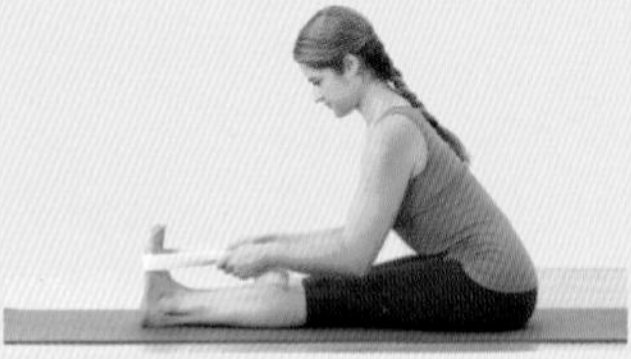

2 Maintaining this posture, stretch your arms up as far as possible. They should lie next to your ears. Hold the hands with open palms forward.

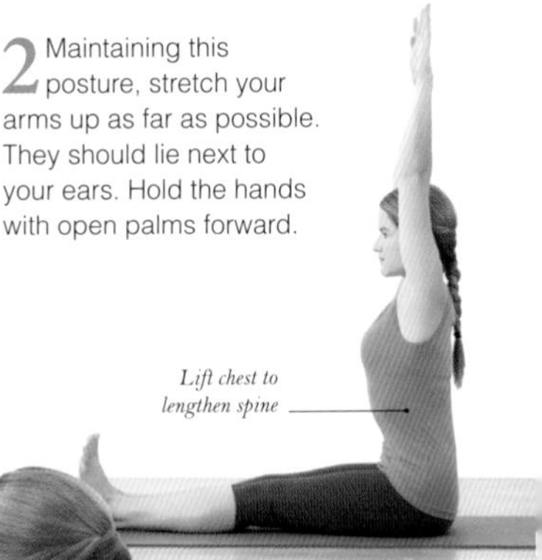

Lift chest to lengthen spine

3 Again, making sure to keep your back straight, lean forward from the waist, and reach for your ankles with straight arms. Hold for a few breaths, then release.

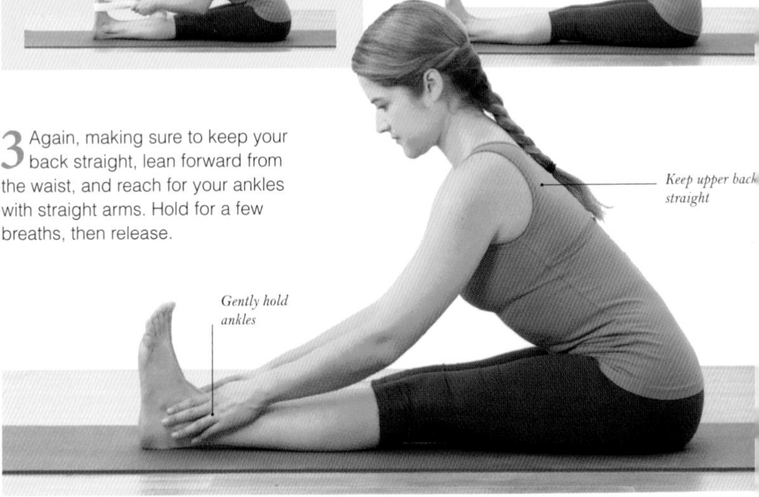

Keep upper back straight

Gently hold ankles

73 SEATED FORWARD BEND VARIATION

If you want a little extra stretch in the hamstrings and lower back, try this more difficult variation on the exercise opposite. The secure grip that the hands take on the toes helps you bring your torso farther over your legs.

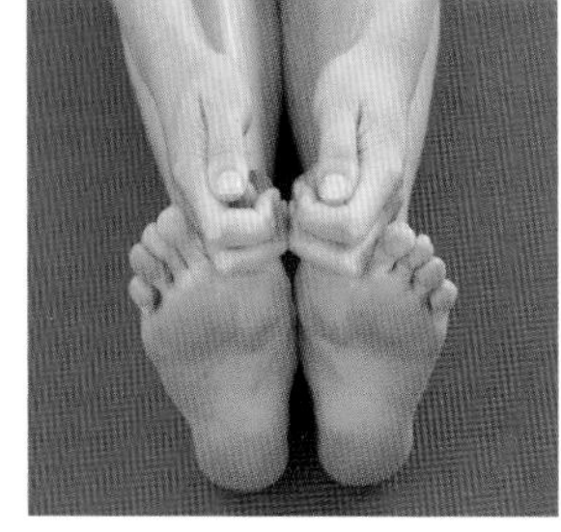

Correct, secure hand positions

Back, neck, and head are aligned
Keep legs lengthened and flat
Lean forward from hips

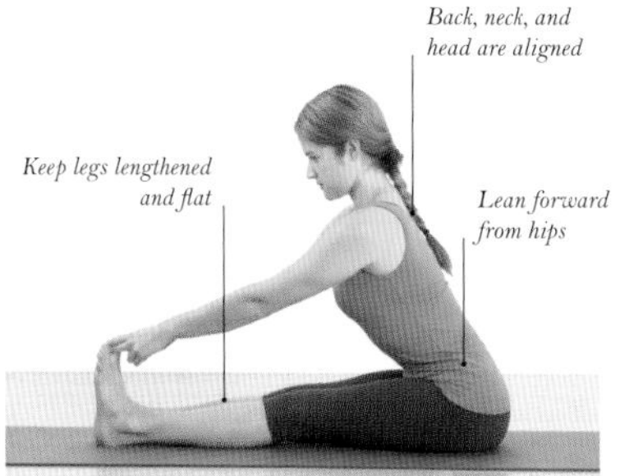

1 Sit with your legs straight out in front of you. On an out breath, bend forward, keeping your back straight and extending your arms. Grasp your big toes with the first two fingers of each hand, as above.

Lengthen spine by lifting through chest

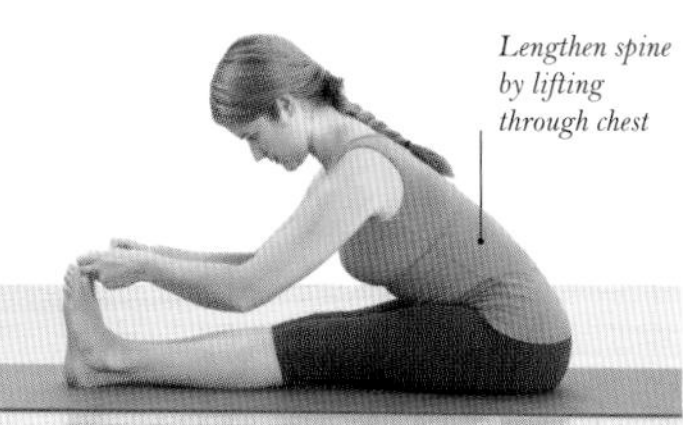

2 Exhaling, bend farther forward to stretch the spine. Bend your elbows so that they help you with the forward movement. Be sure to keep your legs straight, and maintain the grip on your toes.

3 Exhale, bending farther so the elbows come to the mat and the abdomen to the thighs. With each out breath, extend more, focusing on your toes.

Extend forward with each breath out
Bring abdomen as close to thighs as possible

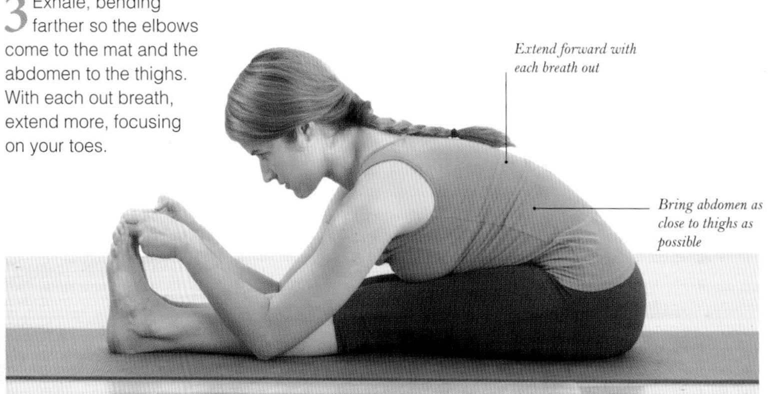

POSES FOR RELAXATION

74 HOW YOGA PROMOTES RELAXATION & HARMONY

The purpose of yoga is to unite all the levels of our being, bringing about harmony of mind, body, and spirit. It serves to nourish the entire body and nervous system, through improved circulation and by balancing hormones, which in turn helps promote relaxation. Breathing exercises and meditation bring about mental and spiritual calm. All these aspects work together to create relaxation and harmony within.

75 COW ARMS

This yoga pose exercises both arms simultaneously, at the same time also enhancing upper-body flexibility and awareness of your own posture.

Clasp fingers securely

Rear view

Keep head centere

Breathe rhythmically

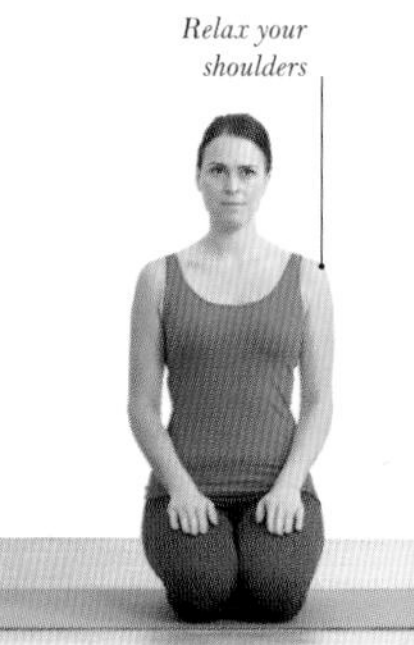

1 Kneel, sitting on your heels, with your toes pointing backward. Look forward and soften the muscles of the face. Relax the shoulders as you breathe.

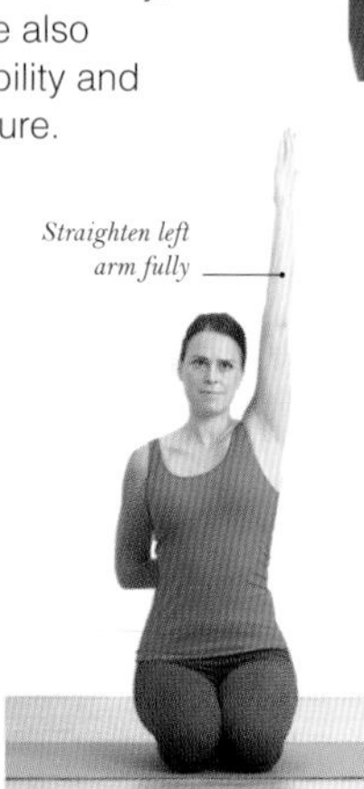

2 Inhale, and raise your left arm up. Work the stretch along the side of your body. Bend your right elbow so that the right hand is on your lower back, palm facing out.

3 Bend your left arm, so the hand is between your shoulders. Push the right arm higher up your back, palm still out, until you can clasp the fingers of both hands together. Pull gently. Exhale to undo, and flick your fingers to release any tension. Switch sides.

76 CHILD'S POSE

This posture offers a useful counter-stretch to backward bends and helps normalize the circulation. The Child's Pose can be used either to prepare for, or recover from, other poses.

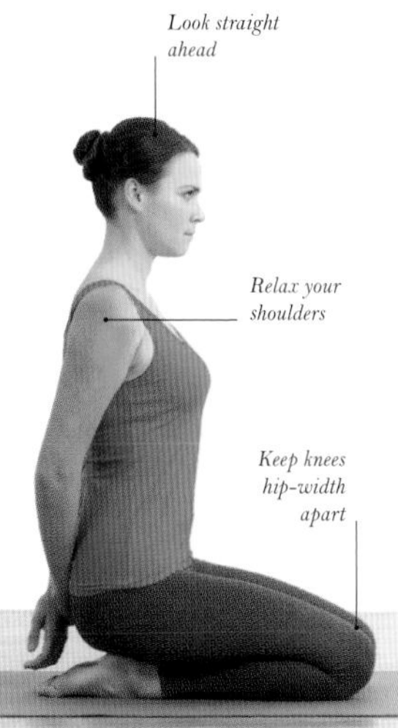

1 Kneel, sitting on your heels, with your big toes touching. Keep your spine straight. Clasp one wrist with the other hand.

Feel breath at back of rib cage
Touch mat with forehead

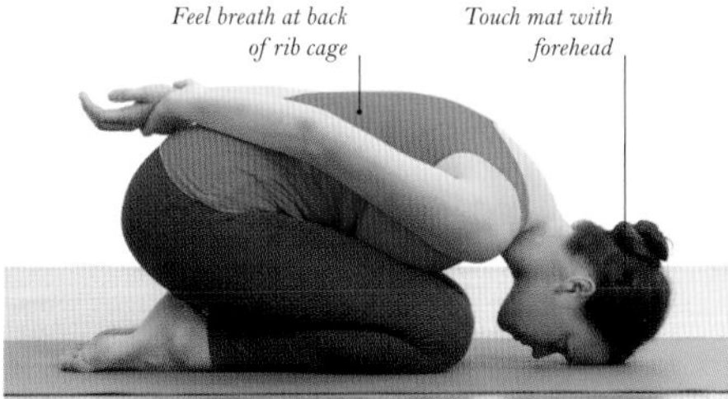

2 Exhaling deeply, slowly move your head and chest down as far as possible, bending from the hips. Continue folding forward until your forehead rests on the mat.

3 Unclasp your hands, and allow them to rest on the floor, palms up. Focus on your breathing. Hold this position for several minutes.

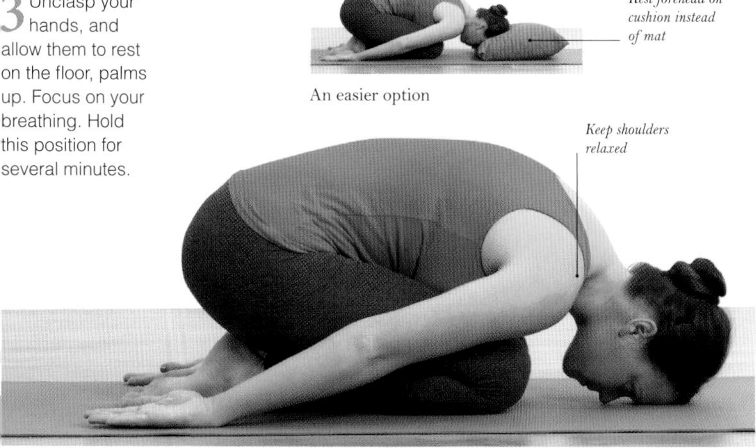

An easier option

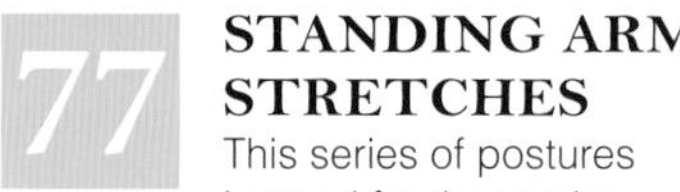

77 STANDING ARM STRETCHES

This series of postures is good for those who wish to improve the harmony between their breathing and movement. It is also valuable for the stretch it gives across the shoulders and along the spine.

Hold clasped hands to sternum
Allow back to curve naturally
Keep feet together

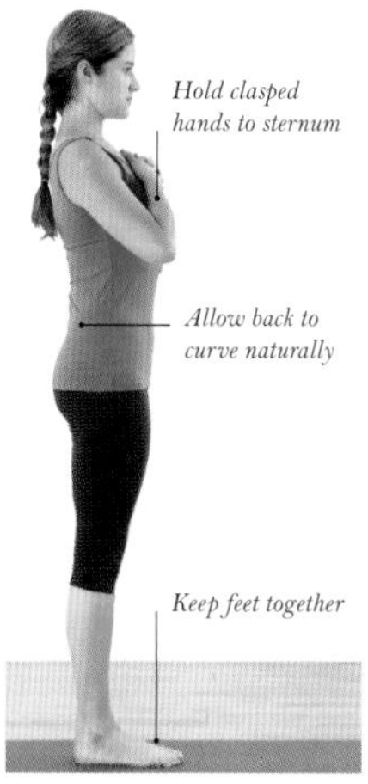

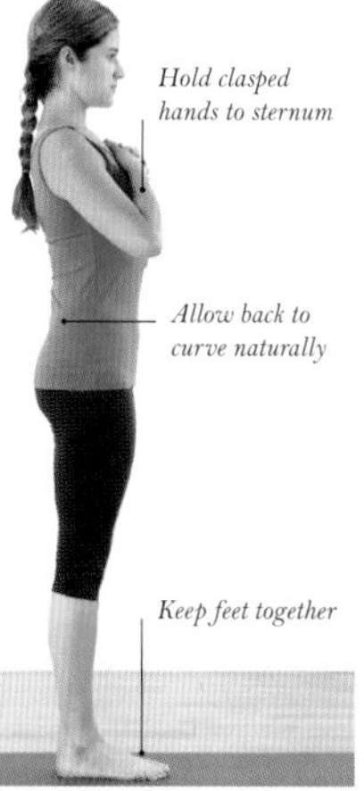

1 Stand with your feet together, and interlock your fingers. Place your hands on your chest, palms down. Feel the movement of your chest as you breathe.

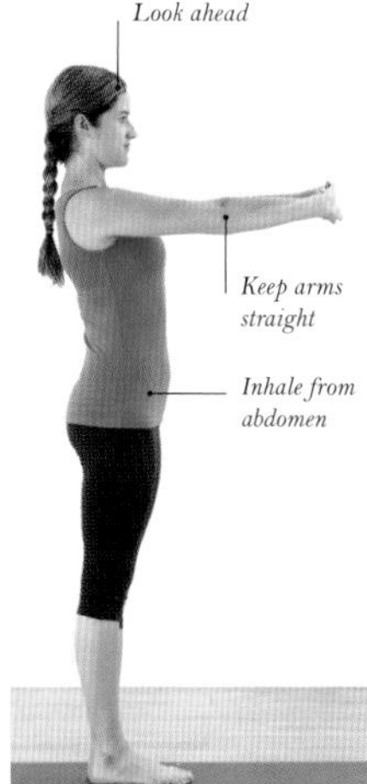

2 Breathe in, stretching out your arms, with fingers interlocked but palms now facing out. Exhale to bring your arms back to your chest.

Lock elbows
Raise arms to 45°
Keep legs straight

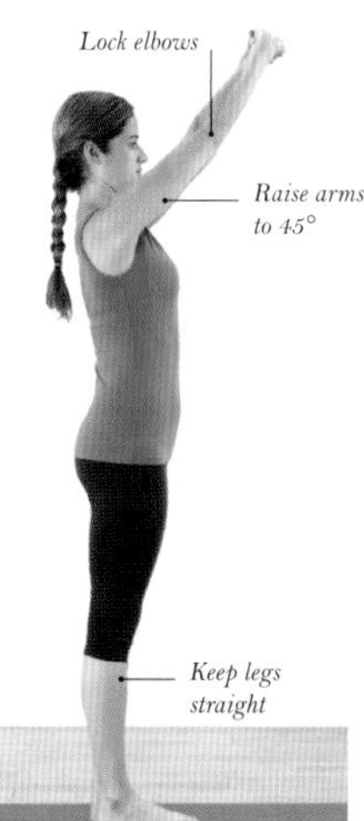

3 Repeat the movement in step 2, but this time extending your arms up at an angle of 45 degrees. Inhale on extension, and exhale on return.

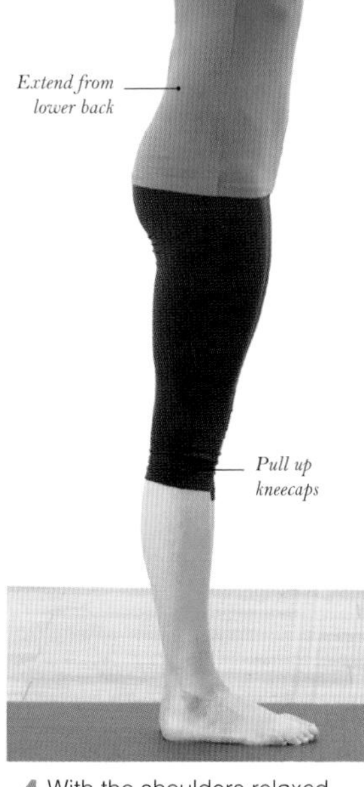

4 With the shoulders relaxed, repeat steps 1 and 2, but this time extending your arms up and lengthening your spine. Exhaling, return to the start position. Do each stretch at least five times.

78 EASY FLOOR TWIST

This exercise is ideal for relieving tension, which it does through stretching and relaxing the spine and legs. The twisting motion across the torso also helps with the detoxification of abdominal organs.

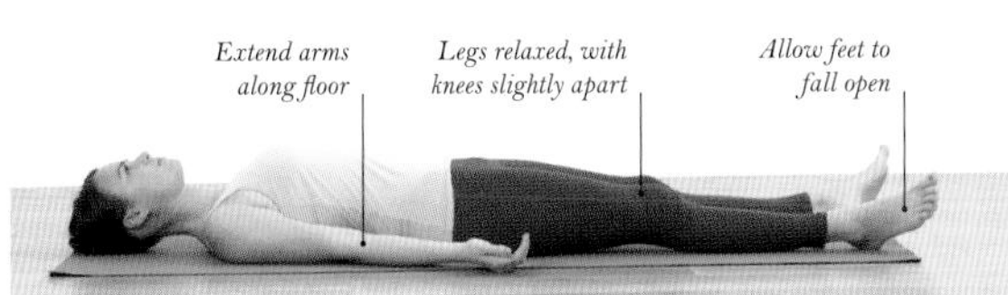

1 Lie flat on your back. Relax your shoulders, and rest your arms beside your body, palms up.

2 Bring your right toes up toward your left knee. Exhale, guiding the right knee over the left leg, with the toes pressing into the left leg. Move the right arm along the floor.

Move arm away from body
Lift right buttock from floor
Push right foot into back of left knee

Turn head to face right
Relax left foot

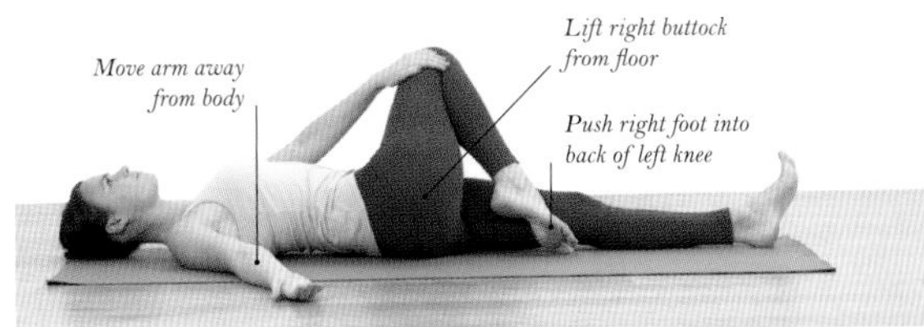

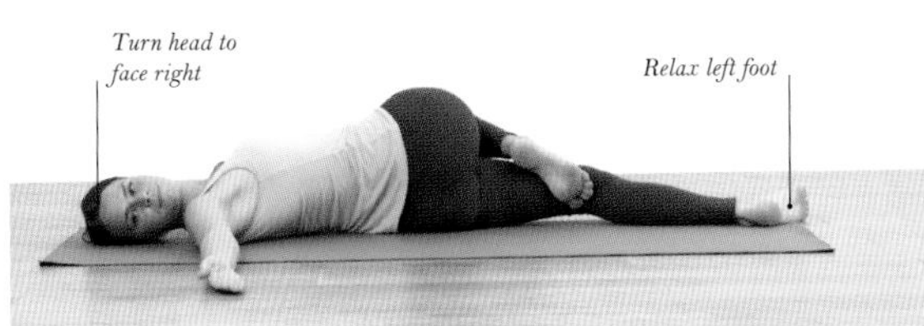

3 Exhale to rotate farther, trying to take your right knee to the floor. Stretch your right arm out at 90 degrees, and turn your head right. Hold for up to ten breaths. Inhale to release.

4 Once back in the starting pose, repeat the exercise, this time bending the left leg. Once completed, inhale and gently reverse the movements.

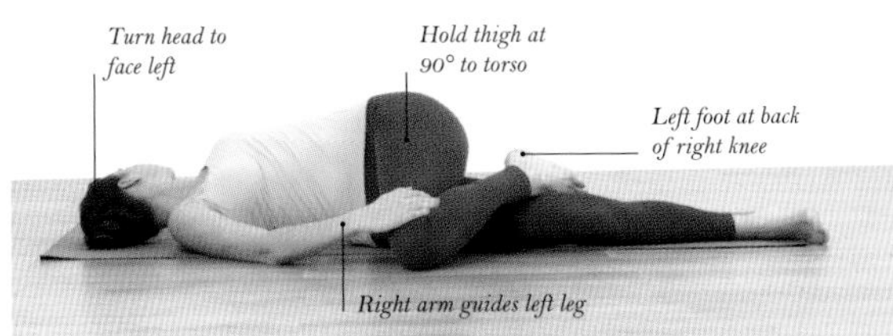

Look straight ahead

Keep your back straight

1 Sit sideways on the chair, with the backrest next to your right arm and your feet on the floor. Place your hands on your thighs, and relax the shoulders.

79 CHAIR TWIST

Spinal twists such as this one are easy, effective ways to bring yoga into your day-to-day routine. The Chair Twist can be practiced anywhere in just a few minutes, as long as you have a chair with a straight back. It is a good exercise for stretching the spine and releasing tension in the neck and shoulders. As with all yoga asanas, perform the exercise on both sides of the body.

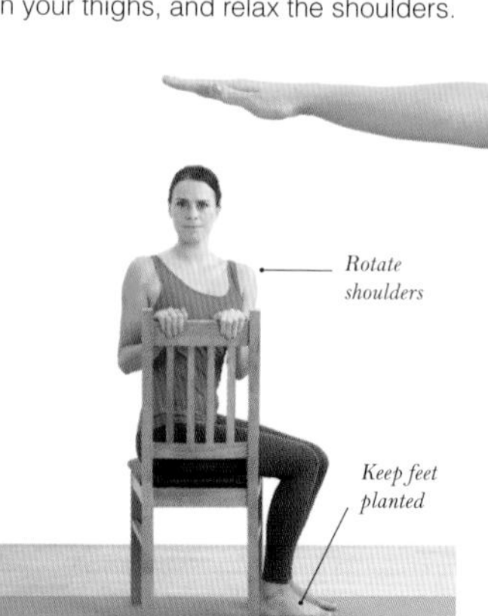

2 Turn right and take the backrest with both hands, inhale, and lift your chest. Exhale, twisting from the lower back toward the rear of the chair.

3 Stretching the spine up, turn the torso, shoulders, neck, and head as far right as is comfortable, and raise your right arm. Hold for several breaths.

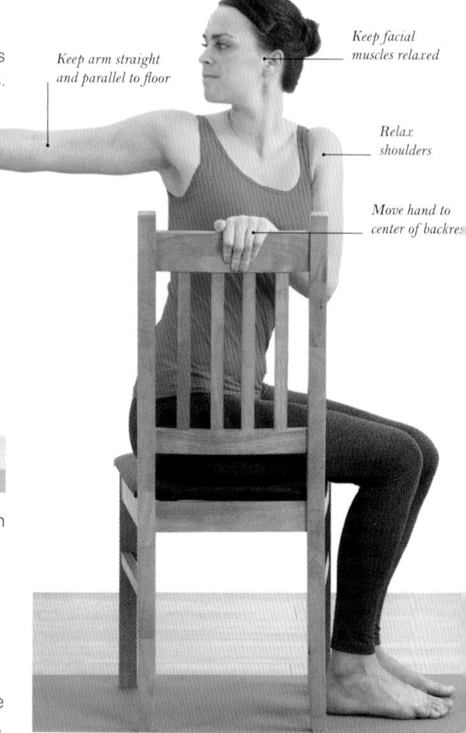

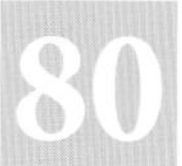

80 CROSSED LEG FORWARD BEND

This pose is beneficial for the practitioner in several ways. Not only does it relieve tension in the lower back but it also improves digestion and helps calm the mind. Additionally, it helps with the opening of the hips and outer thighs.

Align head to neck and back
Elongate your spine, keeping it straight throughout
Pull knees down
Place palms in front of you

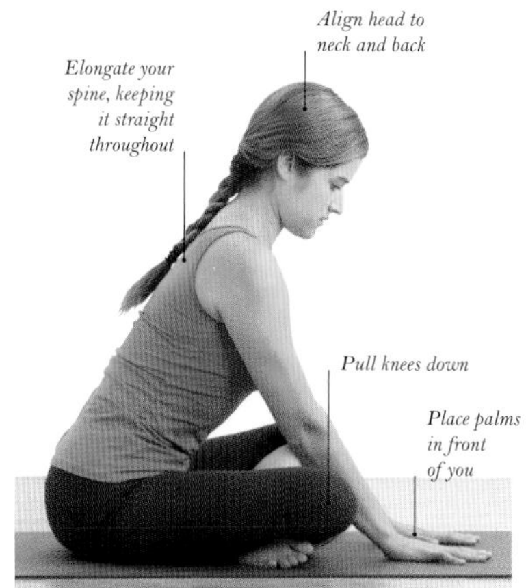

THINGS TO REMEMBER

When you are attempting to move your head closer to the floor, you may find that the front foot slips forward. Counter this by sitting on a blanket, but with your feet on the mat. Be careful not to pull from the neck when you are lowering your head. The back, neck, and head should remain aligned, and you should keep your back straight throughout the entire exercise.

1 Sit cross-legged and well rooted, with your right ankle in front of the left. Hinge forward from the waist, setting your palms on the floor. Exhale and lean forward.

2 Pushing down through your tailbone, stretch your torso and arms, moving your palms farther forward. As you exhale, try to move farther still. Hold for five to ten breaths before releasing.

Keep shoulders relaxed
Look down toward hands
Root down through tailbone
Straighten your arms

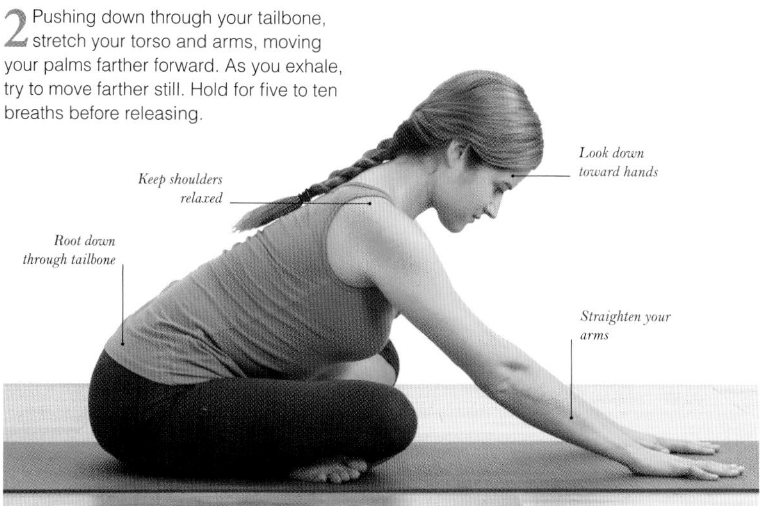

POSES FOR BALANCE

81 HOW YOGA IMPROVES BALANCE

Asanas and breathing exercises help build core and overall muscular strength and flexibility. They also improve reflex responses while developing a calm, focused mind and profound bodily awareness. This all leads to better balance and poise, both physically and mentally. Balance is improved by working the body through a range of different postures. With consistent, mindful yoga practice, the body gradually becomes better poised. Combine your practice with meditation to balance yourself mentally as well as physically.

82 TREE POSE

This pose helps aid balance through concentration, by building strength and flexibility in the leg muscles. Start standing with the feet together, and inhale as you transfer your body weight onto your left foot.

Keep rib cage lengthened
Place right foot high up left leg
Feel chest opening

Pull abdomen in toward spine
Keep standing leg straight and firm

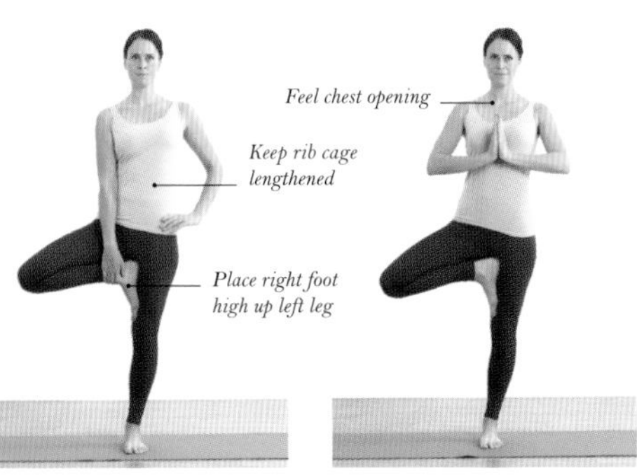

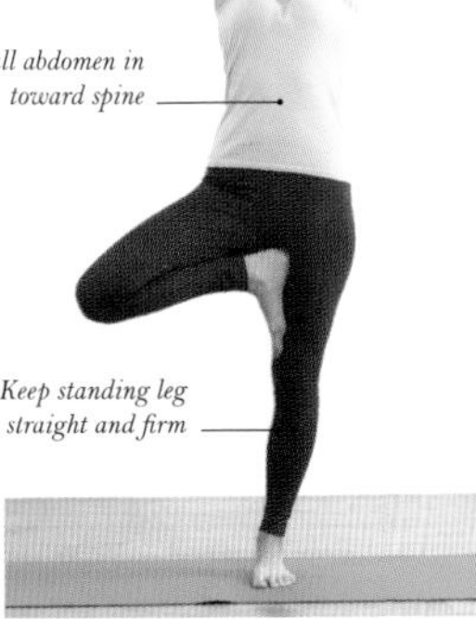

1 Bend the right knee and place your right foot on the inside of the left leg, using your right hand to position it as high as is comfortable.

2 Push down through your left leg and breathe deeply, finding your point of balance. Inhale, and bring your hands to the prayer pose.

3 Fix your gaze straight ahead and, inhaling, extend your arms up, touching your palms together. Take a complete breath, then come out of the pose and repeat on the other side.

83 HALF LOTUS TREE

This hip-opening, standing posture requires you to use not strength but concentration and balancing skills.

1 Start with your feet together, and breathe in to transfer your weight to the right foot. Bend the left knee and raise the left foot. Draw your left foot as high up the right leg as you can.

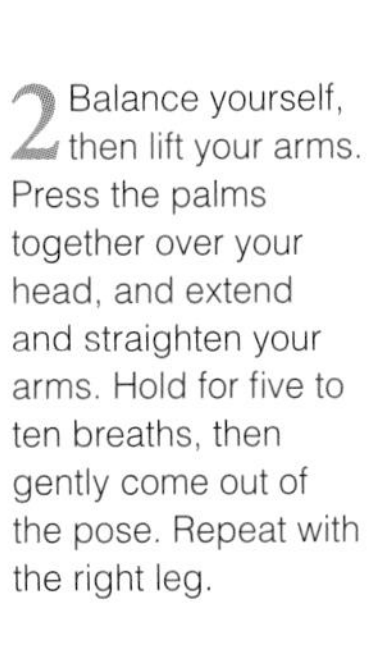

2 Balance yourself, then lift your arms. Press the palms together over your head, and extend and straighten your arms. Hold for five to ten breaths, then gently come out of the pose. Repeat with the right leg.

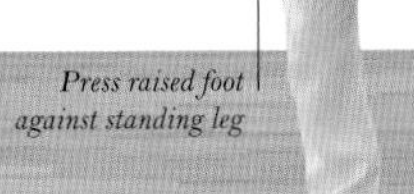

84 EAGLE

This asana helps strengthen the core and so promotes centering and alignment. The joints are nourished by increased blood flow.

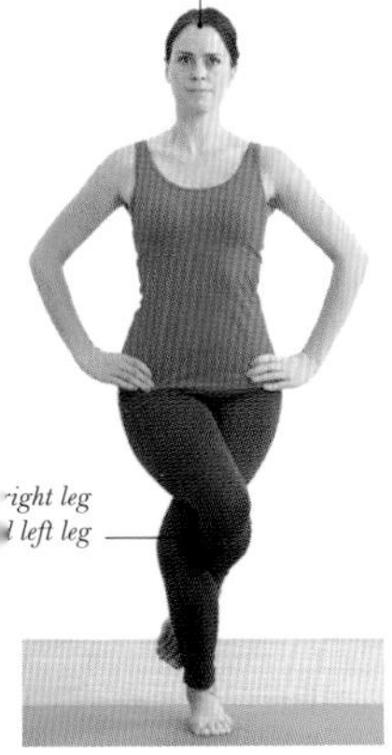

1 From a standing pose, bend your knees slightly and balance on the left foot. Cross the right thigh over your left, hooking the right foot behind it.

2 Lift your arms with the elbows bent. Wrap your right arm and hand under and around the left, pressing the palms together. Repeat on the right.

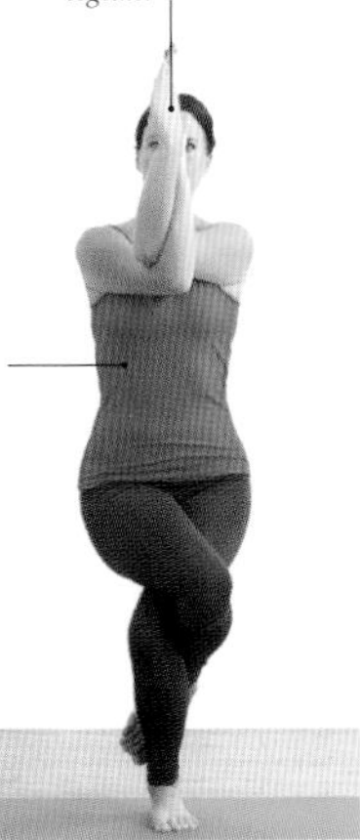

85 HALF SHOULDER STAND WITH WALL

Inverted asanas reverse the direction of blood flow, increasing the supply of blood to the face and brain, as well as to the heart and other organs. Such postures are particularly restorative. This pose is good for improving circulation.

Straight legs, supported by wall

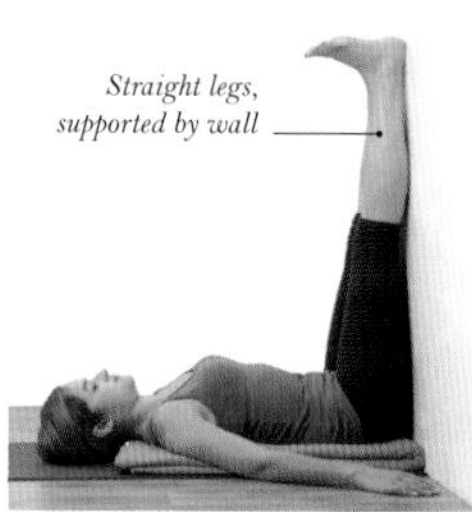

1 Place your mat at right angles to the wall. Put a folded blanket on top of it, with the fold next to the wall. Follow steps 1–3 of Tip 65, but end with your palms flat on the floor, next to the mat.

Keep thighs slightly angled
Stabilize yourself by pushing your feet into the wall
Raise torso away from wall
Use hands to support your back

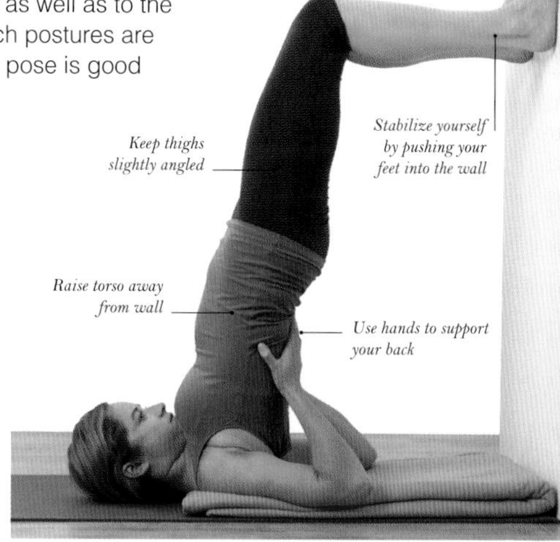

2 Bend your knees, so your feet are flat to the wall and shins parallel to the floor. Pushing off from your feet, raise your torso and place your hands on the small of your back.

Point left foot
Keep leg straight
Support weight with hands

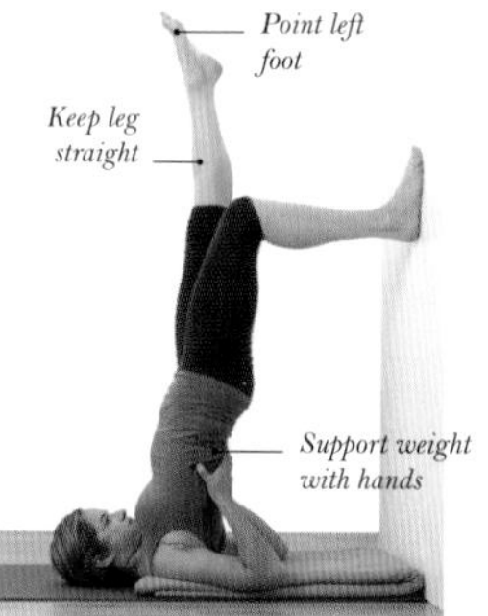

3 Take the time to carefully adjust your position, with the aim of making your back as straight as possible. Then take the left leg from the wall and point it straight up.

Point both feet
Align knees to hips
Hold torso straight

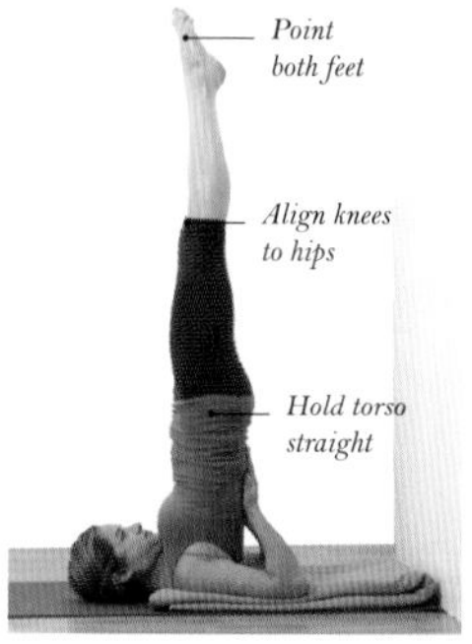

4 Bring your right leg beside the left, adjusting your hands for extra support. Breathe. Reverse the steps until you are on your back with legs up the wall.

Roll over by rotating along lower back

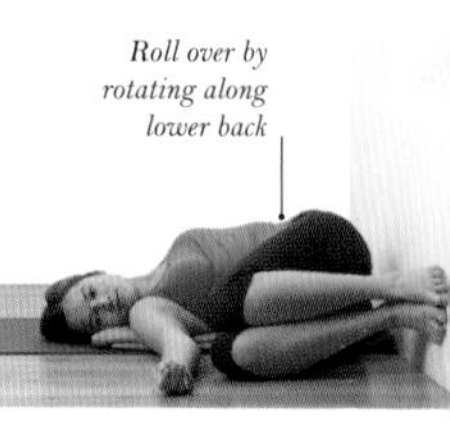

5 As you exhale, bend your knees over the chest. Gently drop the legs sideways until your knees reach the floor. Rest for a few breaths, then sit up.

86

CAT BALANCE

Quite a lot of the yoga postures that are good for balance tend to start from a standing position. However, Cat Balance begins on the floor. Practice this asana to develop your core and strengthen your arms and legs. Repeat each step five times, alternating limbs.

Keep back flattened

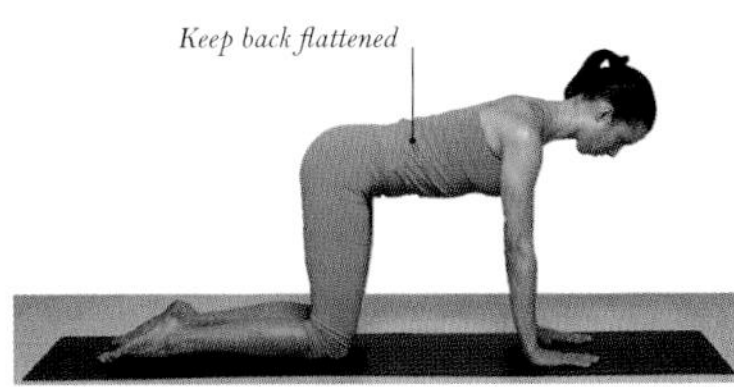

1 Position yourself on all fours, with wrists directly below the shoulders and knees under the hips. Point your toes. Draw your navel toward the spine to flatten your back.

Arm should be in line with ear
Draw tailbone back
Hold raised arm straight

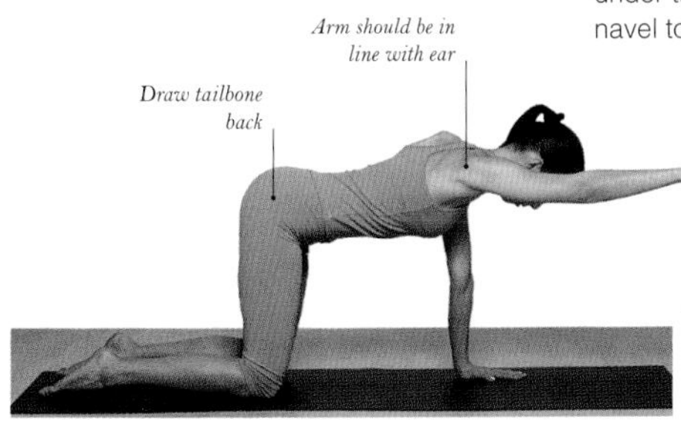

2 Inhale and raise your right arm while tightening the abdominal muscles. Keep your arm in line with the body. Exhale to lower the arm. Repeat with the left arm.

Keep raised leg as straight as you can
Back is held straight

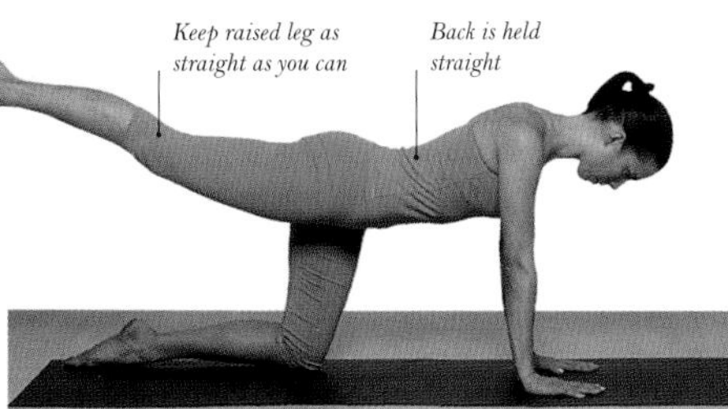

3 Return to the starting pose. Inhale and pull in the abdomen as you raise and stretch your right leg, aligning it to your shoulders. Lower your leg as you exhale.

4 Return to your starting position. On the in breath, extend your left leg and right arm at the same time. Hold for five breaths.

Keep hips level
Point toes
Spread fingers to help support body weight

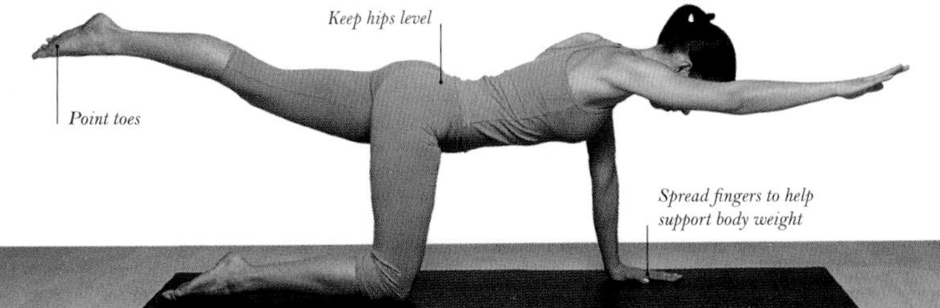

THE COOL-DOWN

87 IMPORTANCE OF THE COOL-DOWN

The cool-down after your yoga practice is an important component of the session, so be sure not to rush or skip it. It will calm your mind and relax your muscles, but it also allows your body to absorb the energy that has been released through the various yoga postures, thereby maximizing the value of the session.

88 PHYSICAL RELAXATION

Assume the Corpse pose (see pp.66–67), then physically tense and relax all the muscles in your body, one body part at a time. Start at the toes and work your way up. Once you have finished, start at the toes again and mentally relax all those same muscles. Last of all, take a few moments to relax your mind.

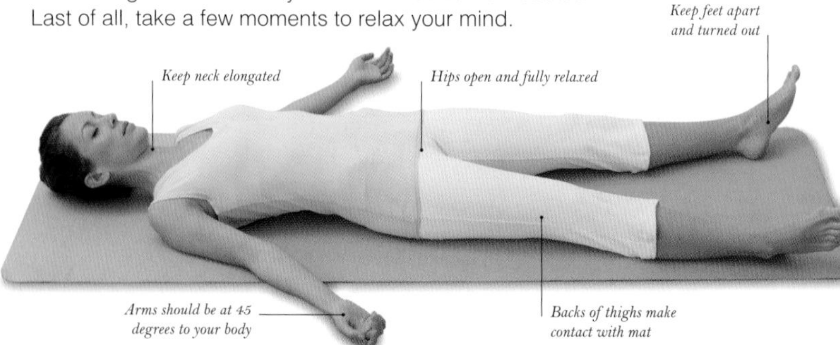

89 MENTAL RELAXATION

The yoga cool-down, or relaxation stage, is more of a mental exercise than a physical one. This is because it requires you to send mental messages to your body parts, instructing them to tense and relax. Once that is done, you finish the cool-down by relaxing your mind, too.

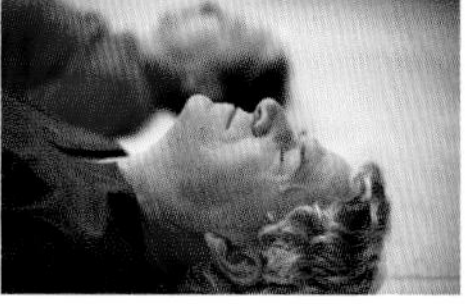

Take time to relax your mind

90 HOW LONG TO RELAX FOR?

Your end-of-session relaxation is based on the Corpse pose, which should also be employed at the beginning of your yoga practice. Relax fully by resting in this position for at least five minutes.

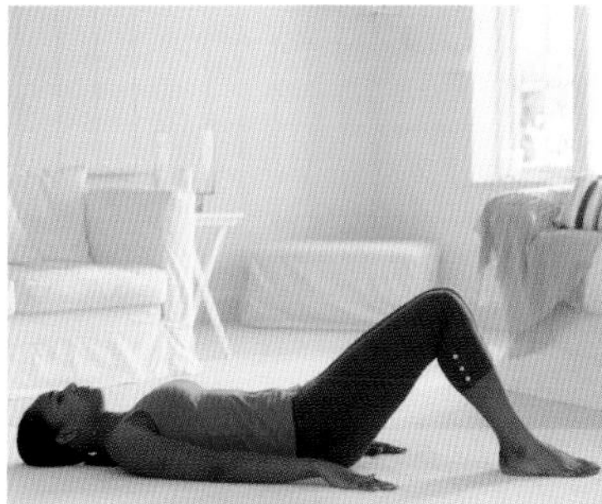

Knees bent, with feet on the ground

91 ENDING YOUR COOL-DOWN

While in Corpse pose, allow your breath to be full and easy. Wiggle the fingers and toes, gradually waking up the body. Bend your knees, keeping your feet on the ground. Draw the knees to your chest, hug them in, and gently roll from side to side. Roll on to one side and push yourself up into a seated position. End by bringing the hands to prayer pose.

92 CUPPING THE EYES

Just as it is important to warm up the eyes before your yoga session (see p.26), you should also take the time to cool them down after your practice.

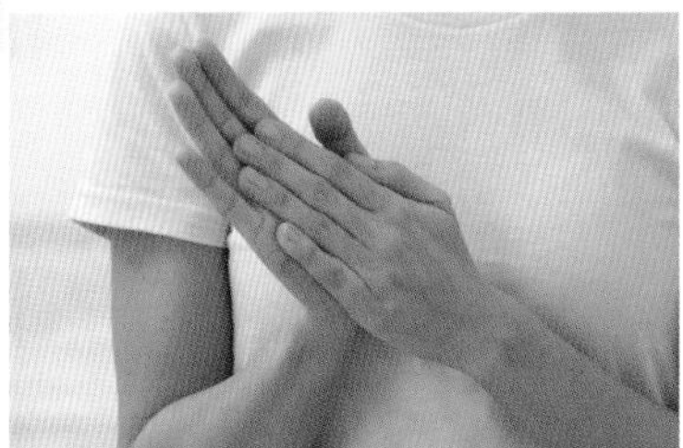

1 Sitting comfortably, with your back straight, rub your hands together until they begin to warm up a little.

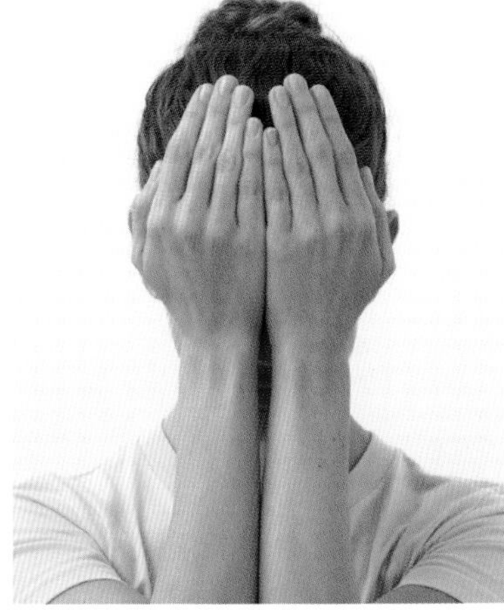

2 Close your eyes. Breathing easily, place your hands over your eyes for several minutes, completely obscuring your vision.

93 IMPORTANCE OF THE CORPSE POSE

The Corpse pose is the ideal way to end your yoga sessions, as well as being a good start to your workouts. It allows the body the time to absorb all of the good muscle and mind work that has been done during your practice time, letting released energy flow freely and expelling waste products from the muscles. It helps you relax in preparation for the rest of your day.

94 CORPSE POSE

In this extended version of the classic Corpse pose, the full length of the body is held in alignment and completely supported by the floor. This allows for deep relaxation in all of the muscles.

1 Lie with knees bent and feet flat on the floor. Interlock your fingers behind your head. Lift the head to look forward toward your knees.

Use hands to assist movement of head
Knees raised and slightly apart

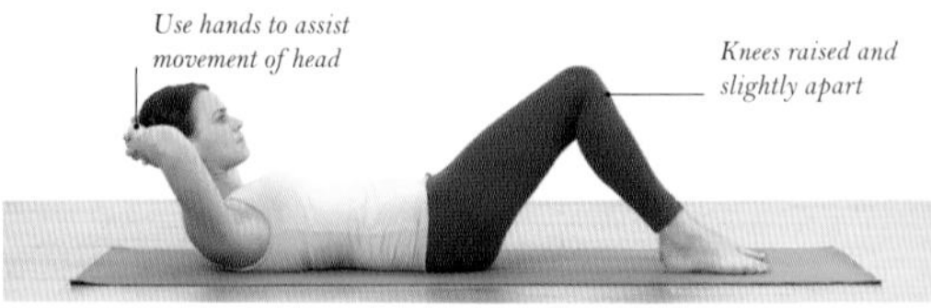

2 Lie fully extended, with eyes closed if you want. Starting from your feet, work up the body, breathing any tightness out of your muscles.

Relax all muscles
Let feet fall outward

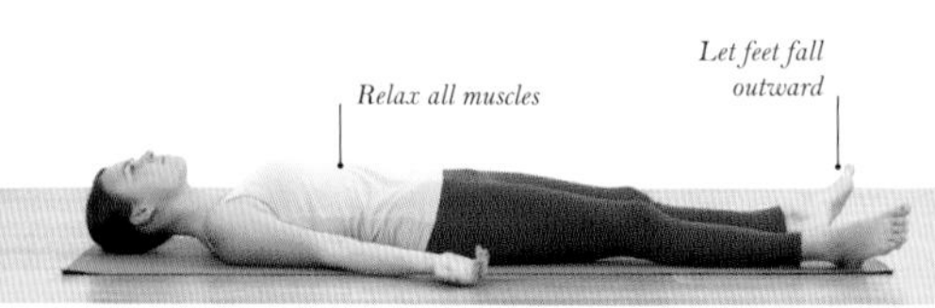

3 Inhale as you raise your right leg by about 1 ft (30 cm). Tense the right leg, keeping everything else relaxed. Hold, then lower and switch legs.

Focus on tension in leg
Hold leg tense for one breath

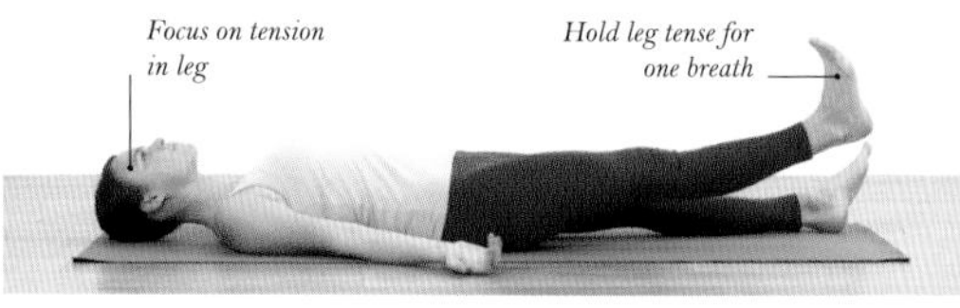

4 Arch the upper back to lift the chest, pulling the shoulder blades in. Keep the head and bottom on the floor. Hold for one breath, then release.

Arch upper back on inhalation
Point toes away

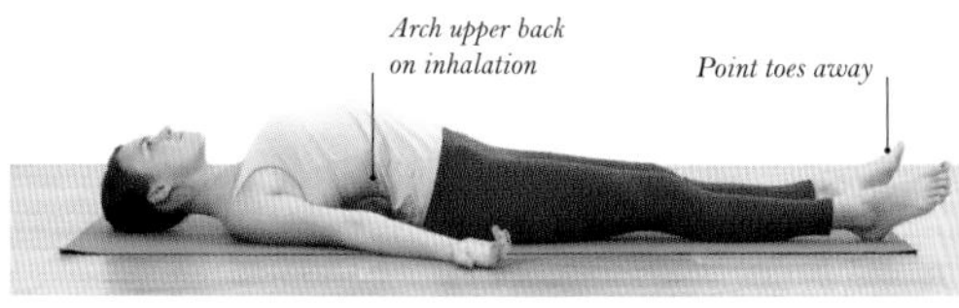

95 CORPSE POSE: ADDITIONAL RELAXATION

The following postures can be tagged on to your Corpse pose relaxation at the end of your yoga session, or you can pick and choose the steps that you think would most benefit you on any given day, focusing on the areas that feel most tense.

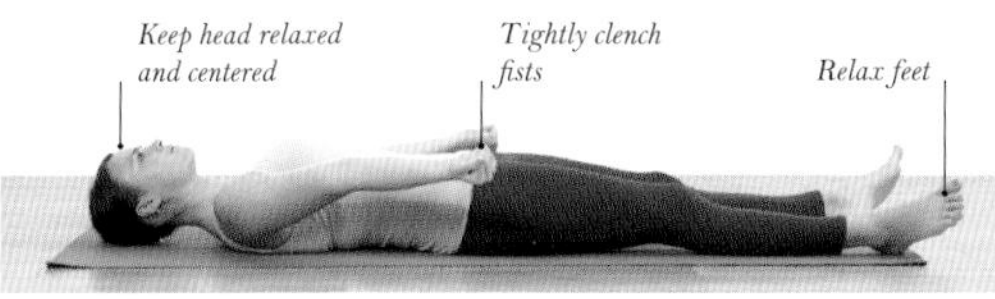

1 Inhale, raising your arms by about 1 ft (30 cm). Tense both arms, making fists with your hands. Hold for one breath, and exhale to lower.

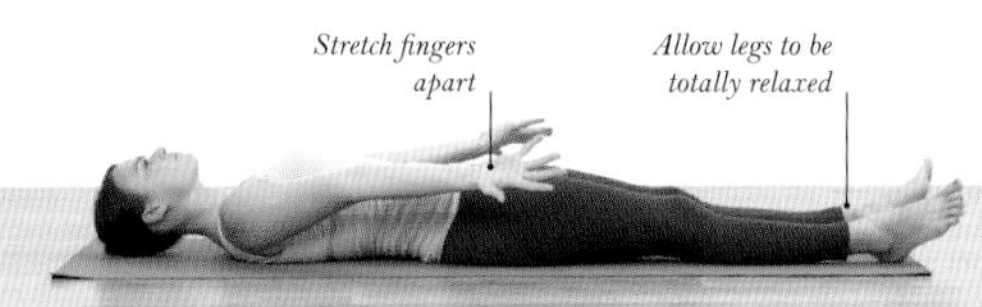

2 Inhale to raise both arms, palms up and fingers apart. Tense your arm muscles. Hold for one breath, then exhale as you take the arms back down.

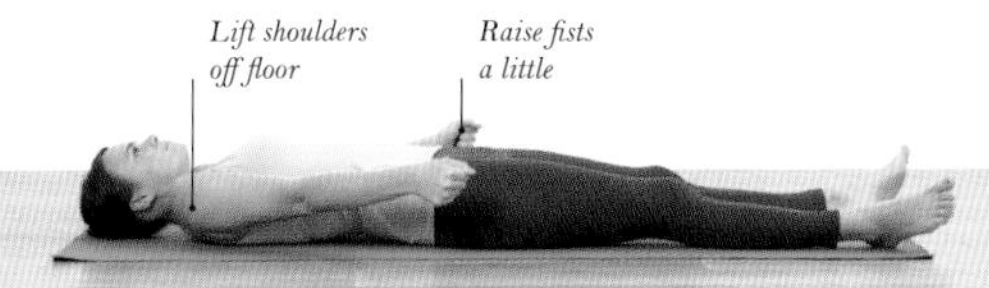

3 Clench your fists and breathe in as you hunch your shoulders up and raise your arms off the floor. Hold for one breath, then exhale to release.

Close eyes if preferred
Keep feet loose and relaxed

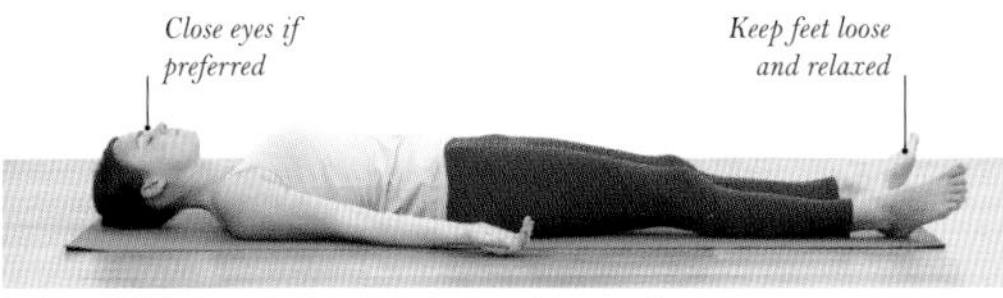

4 Lie completely relaxed. Free your mind of all concerns. Each time you breathe out, focus on the tension leaving your body. Rest for a few minutes.

Support head with hands
Stack legs one on top of the other

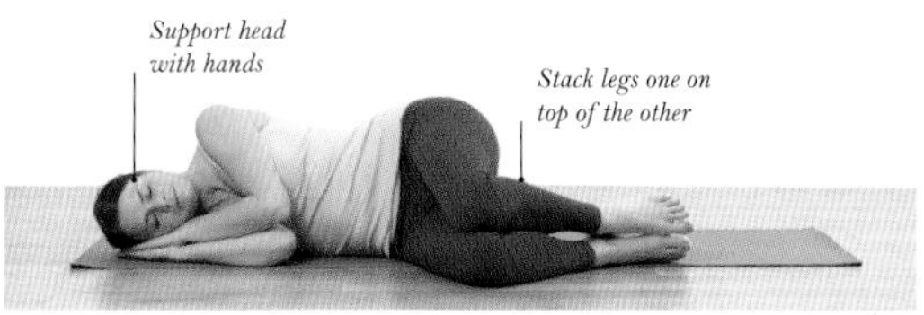

5 At the end of your relaxation, bend your knees and roll to one side. Rest a while, then use the hands to push the upper body off the floor and into a kneeling position.

96 USING MEDITATION

Although meditation is perfectly suited to everyone, it is particularly beneficial for those who have busy lives, either because of stressful jobs or because of a vast array of family and household commitments. Meditation helps calm the overactive mind, thereby reenergizing you, increasing your stamina, and improving your powers of concentration. Through the regular use of meditation, it is within your grasp to create a sense of inner peace and have a clear mind.

WHAT IS MEDITATION?

A good way to grasp the real essence of true meditation is to consider a lake. Think about how you can clearly see the bottom of the lake when the surface is still. However, when there are a lot of waves, you are unable to see much below the surface at all. This is the perfect analogy for the mind: when your mind is still, you are better able to experience inner calm.

98 WHERE & WHEN TO MEDITATE

You are free to meditate wherever you are comfortable, but there are some considerations to bear in mind. If you choose to meditate indoors, pick a room that is warm, clutter-free, and away from distracting noises. If you go outside, find somewhere with as little activity as possible but where you are safe and able to relax fully. Meditation can be practiced at any time of day or night, but it is easier to train your mind if you are able to set a regular time slot.

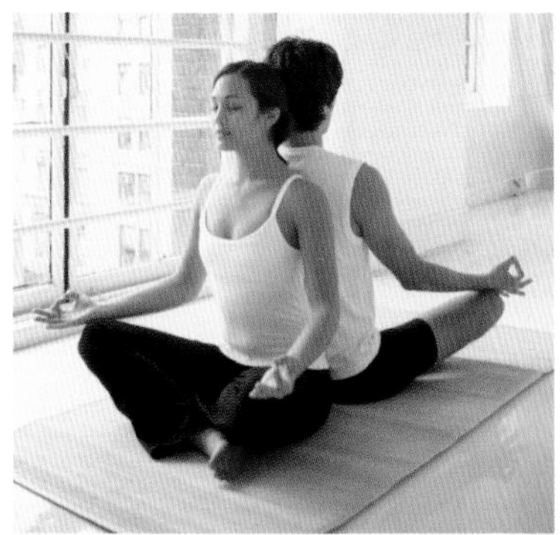

MEDITATING TOGETHER
You do not have to meditate alone. It can be done in pairs or even in larger groups. Mass meditations are often held around the world.

MEDITATION POSITION

To allow yourself to meditate correctly without any distractions it is important to take a comfortable sitting pose. Your legs should be crossed, and your spine should be straight. Keep your shoulders straight but relaxed. This is an easy, natural pose for children, but adults may require some assistance. If you feel any tension in your lower back, try sitting on the front edge of a cushion.

Keep shoulders straight but relaxed
Focus your mind

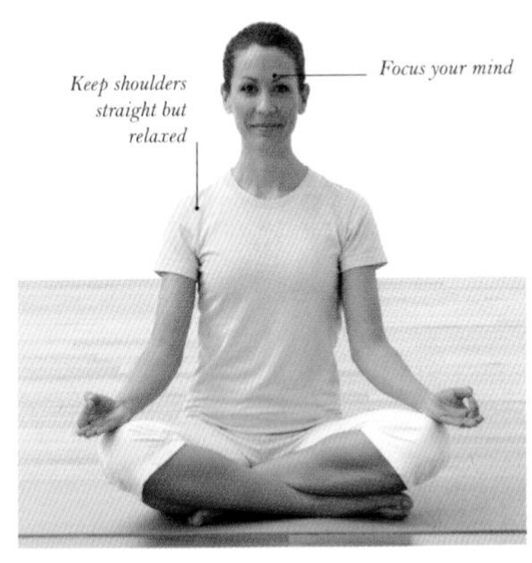

YOGIC BREATHING

Correct breathing is a key part of meditation and concentration. First, oxygenate your brain with 5 minutes of deep abdominal breathing. Next, slow down but still breathe rhythmically, in for 3 seconds, then out for 3 seconds.

Feel chest rise and fall
Start with deep abdominal breaths

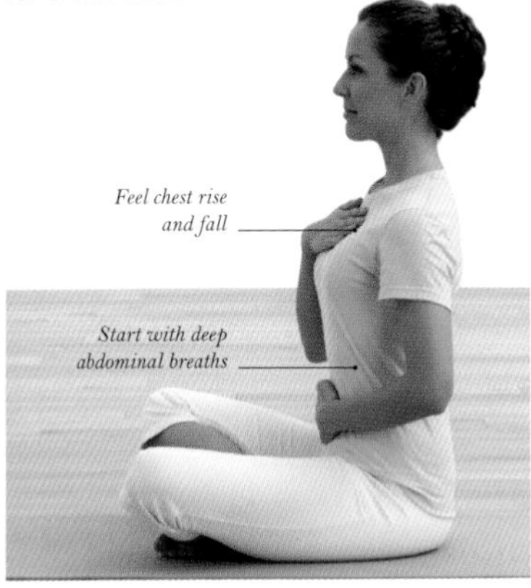

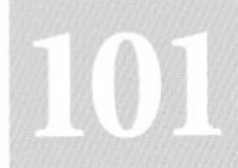

HAND POSITIONS

The hand positions shown below are all used in meditation. Make your hands as comfortable as you can; this helps you relax. Resting your hands on your knees or in your lap also helps keep the back and shoulders straight.

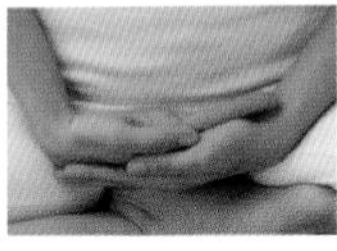

HANDS CUPPED
Place one hand on top of the other, palms up, and place them in your lap.

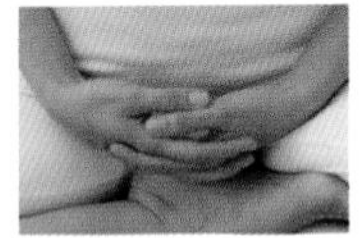

HANDS CLASPED
Interlock your fingers gently, and lay your hands in your lap.

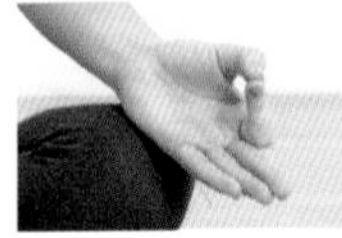

CHIN MUDRA
Form a circle from your thumb and index finger, and rest the hands on your knees.

INDEX

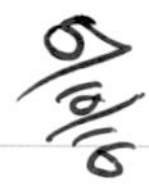

ACKNOWLEDGMENTS

The techniques, ideas, and suggestions presented in this book are intended to provide helpful information and are not meant as a substitute for the advice of a health-care professional. The author and publisher assume no responsibility for any injuries suffered following the practice outlined in this book and specifically disclaim any responsibility for any liability, loss, or risk, personal or otherwise, that is incurred as a consequence, directly or indirectly, of the use and application of any of the contents of this book.

Sands Publishing Solutions would like to thank
Poggy Hatton for her efficient consultancy work during the project,
as well as for her assistance in fine-tuning the contents at the outset;
Natalie Godwin for design assistance; and the ever-brilliant Hilary Bird
for making such swift work of the index.

Dorling Kindersley would like to thank the following photographers:
Vanessa Davies, Guy Drayton, John Freeman, Steve Gorton, Sian Irvine,
Ruth Jenkinson, Dave King, Kellie Walsh, and Colin Walton.